Other books by Robert Neeves:

Lifestyle Fitness

Lifestyle Fitness II

All Good

ROBERT NEEVES

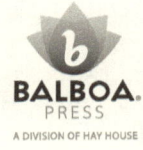

BALBOA.
PRESS

A DIVISION OF HAY HOUSE

Balboa Press books may be ordered through booksellers or by contacting:

Balboa Press
A Division of Hay House
1663 Liberty Drive
Bloomington, IN 47403
www.balboapress.com.au
1 (877) 407-4847

Print information available on the last page.

ISBN: 978-1-5043-0751-2 (sc)
ISBN: 978-1-5043-0755-0 (e)

Balboa Press rev. date: 04/03/2017

No pain, no gain—rubbish!

This book, *Lifestyle Fitness Number Two: All Good*, is all about motivating you to develop a fit and natural-looking body so you can enjoy a full life and fulfil your dreams and expectations. You will not find any crazy, radical diets, which are not only unsustainable but can do more harm than good. You will not find any extreme exercise routines, which only suit a small percentage of the population. Rather, you will find common-sense advice that will help the mainstream, average person to improve and enjoy all aspects of life.

Work, rest, and play: I want you to enjoy the journey as well as the results.

Contents

Acknowledgements

I would like to thank my wife, Trish, for sitting at the computer as she did with my last book, for many hours turning my handwritten scribble into the finished work. I would also like to thank my son, John, and my daughter, Nicole, for assisting with the exercise images.

About the Author

I am an active seventy-two-year-young male. I still enjoy a hard game of squash, and I exercise most days of the week. I am a personal trainer who qualified at the age of sixty-seven in a class of much younger trainees. At the same time, I am not a fitness fanatic. I do not run marathons or participate in triathlons. The human body, I do believe, was not designed for these extreme events; indeed, I believe that they punish our bodies too much. I am not a vegetarian; occasionally I do eat red meat, although my preference is for poultry and seafood. I have nothing against red meat; I simply gave up eating it thirty years ago when the cuts of red meat were not the lean cuts we get today, and I simply never regained my taste for red meat again. I regularly enjoy several beers, which I find give me the relaxation I need, as I tend to be a little over active at times, but I am not suggesting you should start drinking alcohol—far from it. I should possibly replace beer with red wine as research has shown it to be better for you in small amounts. I guess my message is this: everything in moderation. Included in this message is moderate exercise at regular intervals. You do not have to be a gym junkie. The benefit of regular activity requiring lots of movement can be enormous and possibly life changing.

Regular, moderate, consistent exercise; sensible, common-sense eating habits; and a strong, positive, motivated mind are, I believe, most beneficial to our well-being and a positive quality of life. And these things increase in importance as we age. I do not set limits on what I can achieve based on my age. I do think age should not be a barrier to achieving your goal, although I believe a healthy body is vital because it is the vehicle that will carry you as you reach for your dreams and expectations. Without it, are you really getting the most out of life and enjoying it to the fullest?

Two years ago I flew to Africa and went trekking in Tanzania. I successfully reached the highest peak of Mount Kilimanjaro. I was twenty-five years older than the next oldest person in our group, but I was always treated as an equal and never felt outside my comfort zone. One group member complimented me when he said, "I only hope I can do what you are doing when I reach your age." And that is exactly what this book is all about. Not all of those in the group had the fitness capabilities or mindset to keep going and achieve their goals. Okay, so it was not Mount Everest, but it was *my* Mount Everest. I guess everyone has a Mount Everest—a challenge that encourages you to push yourself a little harder, even to your limits. When you achieve the goal, the satisfaction can last the rest of your life. I, like most people, go through life regretting things I have done which I cannot change. I try not to dwell or linger over my thoughts for long, as life is too short. The worst regret for me would be not doing something I wanted to do, should have done, would have done, could have done—but did not.

At the age of nineteen, I was rejected by doctors as being unfit for National Service in the army due to a heart murmur. If I had been passed as fit to serve, I most likely would have been sent to serve in the Vietnam War. I was fully prepared to do my duty as this particular war, in the early stages, was considered to be the right thing, and the dangers were unknown. In hindsight, I realise that my childhood misfortune of contracting rheumatic fever may have been my adult saviour, as that terrible war left a lot servicemen mentally and physically scared.

I still remember going for my military medical. It was like a production line. We moved from one room to another, each room with a different doctor, a specialist in a particular field: eyes, ears, etc. I passed all the tests until I was examined by the heart specialist. A very stern doctor sat behind a large desk reading my induction form. He said, "You have ticked the box which indicates you suffered from rheumatic fever at a young age." When I answered yes, he said in a very unbelieving tone, "Well then, we shall soon see about that, young man." Five minutes later, after checking my chest and back with his stethoscope, his mood changed, and in a much kinder voice, he told me that I could go home. No more tests were required.

I believe living a happy healthy fulfilled life is about balance between activity, rest, and sensible eating habits. It's also about living your life with purpose and not depending on others to make you happy.

I am a registered exercise professional with Fitness Australia (registration number 058426). My specializations include: gym instructor, personal trainer, older adults trainer, and children's trainer.

My "Big Four" for optimal health:

Engage in some sort of regular activity.

All movement is good—the more the better! Doing something—anything—is better than sitting on the lounge for extended periods. Do an activity you like: walking, swimming, riding a bike, exercising, playing games, and so forth. As long as you move your body, just do something. Ideally, your movement should, on occasion, require enough effort to increase your heart rate. Regular enjoyable activity that keeps your body in motion and challenges your abilities is critical to your body and mind for maintaining optimal health.

Indulge in a bit of rest (or inactivity).

Plenty of quality rest will help you stay refreshed and remain calm and tranquil. Simplify your life as much as possible. Try to reduce or eliminate stress. Stress and lack of sleep—or poor quality sleep—go hand in hand. Your body has the time to repair itself while you are resting and sleeping.

Adopt and maintain sensible eating habits.

Nutrition is very important to your health. Whenever possible, eat "real food"—as natural as possible. Include a balanced intake of animal produce, grains, fruits, and vegetables. For the animal produce, fish is best, followed by poultry. I recommend eating less red meat and replacing it with low fat dairy also eggs, nuts and beans are great. Limit your intake of highly processed and fast food. Don't add sugar or salt, as the average person's diet already contains more than we need. Never eat because you are bored. If you are an emotional eater who requires "comfort food," stop for a few minutes and think, *Do I really need this? Is it going to change anything or make it worse?* Instead of eating, go for a walk, clear your head, and relax.

Lead a purposeful life.

Give your life purpose: have an aim in life so you can achieve what you want to. Regardless of your age, look forward to accomplishing something worthwhile. It does not have to be something big: it can be something as small as helping a friend or a stranger. It will give you a great feeling of self-worth.

Great satisfaction and fulfilment are accomplished when you put others before yourself.

Introduction

If you read my first book, *Lifestyle Fitness*, I thank you! This book, *Lifestyle Fitness Number Two*, will move you on with more information, encouragement, and motivation as you take action to improve the quality of your life. It will also summarise, add to, and highlight key sections of my first book that I consider important and worth a review. I also hope it will act as a reminder to keep you on the right track.

Recently I was watching a documentary on television which was shot in the 1960s. It showed a footpath crowd scene in a large American city, possibly New York although it could just as easily been any major city in the developed world—Paris, London, or my hometown, Sydney, Australia. I noticed that everyone in the scene was of a thin build. If we were to watch a similar scene today, most people in the shot would be carrying more weight than necessary, and some would weigh in at dangerous levels.

Today, as I look back on my childhood, I realise that, if someone in our neighbourhood was overweight, he or she would stand out. It was also unusual to see overweight people at school, in the workplace, or just in general. Now the carrying of extra weight has become commonplace, and people have become to accept it as normal. Worse, it seems acceptable, where in reality it is dangerous to our general health and well-being. Being overweight lowers our quality of life and can ultimately lead to a premature death. Most of us have yet to turn the corner, but the average person's weight is increasing at an alarming rate. I find this seriously worrying. It is a major health concern, not to mention a cost to the community, a cost that is increasing as our waistlines increase.

The problem is not only the fat you can see in the mirror; it is also the deposits of fat around your major organs. It is the hidden effects of obesity you cannot see that are the consequences of too much food, the wrong kinds of food, and a lack of exercise. Perhaps some think "out of sight out of mind," but the health risks are real and do exist. Not being able to fit into your favourite jeans may be the least of your problems. If you are overweight and not worried about it, you should be, as it is a growing modern-day problem—growing in size and number. Not only has the number of overweight people increased, the average size of overweight or obese people has increased, and this compounds the problem.

If this scares the life out of you, it is meant to! Please be scared. Do not make the assumption or live under the illusion that everything will be okay. It won't, and I am deadly serious. You have to find a place in your life for physical activity. Your fitness routine should be built into your lifestyle and not an afterthought or add-on. Without good health it is hard to enjoy life. Do not shorten your life with self-inflicted health problems such as type-two diabetes, heart problems, and other challenges brought on by lack of activity and poor eating choices. These afflictions are easily preventable with more activity and healthy eating habits that will reduce your weight and make life much more enjoyable. You have to accept the reality of the situation. Be self-empowered. You control the input of food and drink along with the output of energy. If you are putting more into your mouth than you need or use, on a regular basis, you have a problem. Yes, it is that simple.

If you are one of the small percentage of people with a medical condition like an underactive thyroid, which makes it difficult to control your weight for everyone else you have no excuse. Living in an unhealthy body shape adds to all the serious problems, including pressure on your joints. I am seventy-two and I am lucky to still be very active with little joint pain. Many of my friends are having hip and knee replacements because their joints are worn out from carrying excess weight for a long period of time. It is like having a cement bag strapped to the front of you for twenty years, and that cannot be good. You probably know lifting weights is good for your bones; that is for sure. So why is excess weight not the same as weight lifting? The difference is that excess body weight is there with you 24/7. Carrying this weight on your body puts pressure on your knee and hip joints while you do everyday things like getting out of a chair or bed, quite often from an awkward position.

When you work with weights in a gym, you are in a controlled situation with good posture and techniques. When you have finished your exercise routine, you leave the weight at the gym.

Here is the big difference explained:

If you are overweight and inactive, your joints are under constant pressure trying to support that extra weight that your body was not designed for, especially if you have weak muscles. And we know that inactivity creates weak muscles. If you are the correct weight and exercise or engage in plenty of activity, you will build and tone your muscles. Your body was designed so that your strong muscles could support your joints.

If you are now at the crossroads:

Choose.

How do you want to transport yourself through life?

1. In an overweight unreliable truck down a dirt road full of potholes

Or

2. In a sleek sports car on a smooth highway?

If you choose the highway, read on.

What has changed, and how can we reverse it?

The answer is simple: we have to move more and eat less. To successfully lose weight, you need to burn more calories than you take in. Stop eating before you feel full, try for a satisfied feeling rather than a full or bloated one, and add extra activities to your daily routine.

In today's world, fast and processed food have become more available, more convenient, and more affordable than ever. Also, with the advancement of modern technology, we are moving less.

For those who grew up in the 1950s and 1960s, fast and processed food were available in Australia only at the local fish-and-chip shop or milk bar, which were equivalent to the American drugstore without the pharmacist. Not every family owned a motor vehicle; we walked or rode a bicycle to and from school, shops, and other destinations. Motor vehicles were equipped with manual gearshifts and didn't have power steering, so the driver's arms and legs got at least some exercise!

Now it seems that everyone over seventeen has a modern-day car. We as children always played outside and only came inside to eat our meals. Modern-day children sit indoors playing video games and watching television. They don't exercise. Today we snack on soft drinks and sweets and many other high-calorie foods, which are easily available. In earlier years, snacks and soft drinks were budgeted for only on special occasions; they weren't always in the kitchen cupboard. We faced less temptation, and we ate more fresh food on a regular basis. That is just a small sample of how we moved more and consumed less.

Animals in the wild store fat for the lean times when food becomes in short supply—winter, drought, floods, and so forth. So their food intake evens itself out. This is nature taking care of itself. Human beings in developed countries do not need to store fat in the good times, as there are no lean times. Yet, we just keep adding to our fat levels, increasing our weight, and endangering our health.

If you suffer from high blood pressure and bad cholesterol, you are possibly over indulging in food and alcohol while not partaking in enough exercise or movement. This could be affecting your overall health and well-being. Your excessively indulgent lifestyle, if continued, could shorten your life or leave you with a poor quality of life. Reversing the situation is not all doom and gloom! In fact, the opposite is true: you will improve your current quality of life and enjoy the experience through more active and engaging activities. Your taste buds will soon adjust to having less sugar, salt, and fat. You will find a new purpose in life.

If you now lead a sedentary lifestyle sitting on the lounge watching television with little other activity and eating out of boredom, you may find it difficult to make exercise a regular habit. To start, you will need mental toughness. The personal rewards, however, make it so worthwhile. It is all about *you*, and *you* control the quality of your future.

Start with a strong mindset and focus on what you *can* do rather than what you *cannot* do. Clearly evaluate your short- and long-term goals. Make an effective decision to reach those goals and the life you want.

You must adjust your state of mind. Live intentionally, do not procrastinate, and direct your actions towards a specific purpose. With intent and commitment, you can start off slow and keep on the go. You can adjust and overcome any unexpected obstacles on you road to what you want to achieve! Do not set yourself a standard in life which is below what you deserve. Change your past mindset and do not get trapped into an "I'll believe it when I see it" attitude. Sure, it will take time, and it will not be easy to achieve results, but with hard work and belief in yourself, you can accomplish what you desire. When you do decide to change your destructive lifestyle behaviour, which has probably been a slow change that has crept in over many years, you are only going to return to the way you were before you changed. It is unlikely that you were born with bad habits, so how impossible can it be to change? Hard and slow? Yes! But possible!

You do not have to be perfect. Just be better than you were before. And if you want to be better than you were yesterday, you have to change what you do today. You must change what you have always done with new, positive, consistent action, or you will always be as you are now.

Why not live and enjoy the best life you possibly can? You get only one chance at it.

Now is the time to turn your life around. Do not create excuses or reasons for not taking the first or next step. Once you start, things will fall into place. Let common sense be your guide. You just can't be average anymore because a large percentage of Mr and Mrs Average are unfortunately overweight.

Procrastination can be overcome.

If you are a habitual procrastinator, avoiding projects or starting and not finishing them, or if you do meaningless things because they are easy, or if you avoid things that are important and worthwhile, you may even be low in confidence and self-esteem. You may not feel sure of your abilities. You may fear failure. If you struggle with motivation, acknowledge it. Don't hide it. This may be your first and most important step.

Try asking a friend for help who may be in the same situation. Look for activities you may enjoy and build them into your daily routine: walk the dog, walk to work if possible, or to the shops. If you are going for a coffee with a friend, see if you can find somewhere that is within walking distance for you both. Start off by not setting your goals too high. Make sure they are clear and achievable. Slowly move forward, conquering small steps and milestones one at a time, and crossing them off your list as you build confidence and self-worth. Dance your own dance to your own rhythm. Don't wait for your body to break down because of bad eating habits and an inactive lifestyle. Your health should be about maintaining a healthy body not fixing problems which could have been avoided. Maintenance is easier and cheaper. Start today. Never say, "I will start tomorrow." That is procrastination in its purest form.

Procrastination can be easily overcome, and I have included strategies in Chapter 4. But first, I want to supply you with a few chapters full of information to show you how easy it can be, and to motivate you towards a better life.

I believe in two great motivational cures for procrastination: One, the fear of losing the healthy body you now know, enjoy, and inhabit, which you also take for granted. Two, a real possibility of developing serious, avoidable health complications and discomfort later in life.

Chapter 1

No Pain No Gain? Rubbish!

All Pain-Free Movement is Good!

If you experience pain during or soreness after a workout, you are possibly doing too much too quickly and not giving your body time to adjust. There will be, of course, a period of adjustment that your long-time inactive body absolutely just has to go through. Or you may be not doing the exercise correctly, or using too heavy a weight. Either will put too much strain on your muscles, which could damage your muscle fibres.

Pain or soreness is not necessarily a good gauge of the effectiveness of your workout. Some people feel they have not accomplished anything unless they feel pain or soreness. I believe pain associated with exercise is not good; you can achieve a great workout without pain during or soreness after by taking it slow. By gradually increasing your muscle strength in small steps, you can work out more often and actually enjoy exercise.

Muscle soreness or pain is caused when your muscles are under stress. A small amount of tightness without pain is not a bad thing, but is less acceptable as we age. You may also experience muscle burn, which some people will refer to as mild pain. This is also okay and is not a bad thing as long as you don't experience sharp pain. Muscle burn means you are working hard; your muscles are becoming fatigued and losing power due to an accumulation of lactic acid. If this does occur, do not worry; it is only temporary. After a little active rest as explained later in Chapter 7, you will be back to normal within no time and with no damage done. Assessing muscle burn can also serve as a good gauge of your fitness level as you move forward: the longer it takes in your fitness session to experience muscle burn, the fitter you are becoming. If you challenge yourself with my great high-intensity interval training (HIIT) routine, and you do not push yourself to feel some mild muscle burn, you are doing yourself an injustice.

If you feel you are not doing too much but still experiencing sore muscles or pain, try extending your dynamic stretching warm-up and your static stretching wind-down. Use a massage roller after a workout. When you apply your own body weight, the rolling action and pressure applied along your muscle fibres will increase circulation and aid in muscle recovery time and soreness. It is simple to use in the privacy of your own home. It can also be used before a walk, a workout, or participating in your chosen sport for added flexibility and range of movement, and as they say, if pain persists see your doctor. It is definitely possible to achieve great results from an exercise program, or increased activity like taking up a sport you enjoy or just going for a walk without trying to push yourself through a pain barrier.

Look at it this way: If you were to tread on a sharp object in bare feet, you may not realise it, but your brain would tell you to stop walking before you do serious damage to yourself. It's the same with strenuous activity. Let your brain be your guide. It is designed to be sensitive to your every need. If you are going to work up a sweat, make it a fun, happy sweat without pain.

Disclaimer

Before starting even a light exercise or weight reducing program, you should consult your healthcare professional, even if you are not overweight and feeling good. You will be putting your body under more stress than usual.

Even though these changes can have great long term benefits you need to rule out any hidden medical problems before you begin.

Chapter 2

Why We Need to Move

I keep a completely open mind as to how we started off being on this planet—a creator (a superior being/god) or evolution. Both theories have merit. And there is the chance we came from another planet. However it happened, you must admit our bodies are miracles of construction, designed to perfection, unless you were unfortunate enough to be born with or suffer from a grievous affliction that you will suffer with for the rest of your life. I cannot possibly begin to imagine how painful and distressing that would be.

The majority of the population is born with perfect bodies, and it must be against God's law, the laws of nature, or whatever other laws are out there, to stuff it up the way a large percentage of the population has done today.

We started with a pristine earth, and we are messing it up with mining and the burning of fossil fuels.

We started with pristine bodies, and we are messing them up with overeating and a lack of physical activity.

I am unsure of a few things, but one thing I am sure of is that our bodies were designed for movement. We could not have possibly survived and arrived at this point in time without a lot of work (movement). We needed a lot of flexibility, strength, and movement to be hunter-gatherers who had to catch animals to eat while avoiding animals who wished to eat them. "Why do I need to move today?" you might ask. Many of us have jobs that require us to sit in front of a computer all day. For entertainment, we have a television with an endless number of channels, Internet shopping, and home delivery. Many of our brick-and-mortar businesses are close by and often open 24/7 so we can buy whatever we need.

All movement is good. Vigorous activity or exercise is even better.

Everybody benefits from movement, regardless of his or her physical abilities, age, or gender. Even if you don't enjoy or are unable to exercise, any physical activity is good, and the benefits gained are impossible to ignore.

If this does not sound like common sense, or if you do not agree that Nature intended for us to move frequently, it is up to me to prove it to you. If you are already converted, you may just need to be motivated more to continue or increase your daily physical activity.

The more you move, the more you gain: movement, activity, and exercise.

Here are some very good reasons to get your body moving:

- **Preventing and restoring bone loss:** This is certainly in the top five of importance. All movement prevents and restores bone loss. If you can add weight-bearing exercise to your normal everyday activities, the rewards are even greater. Keeping your bones healthy can prevent and even help reverse osteoporosis. It is never too late, and if that in itself is not enough reason to convince you, there is a heap more.

- **Weight loss:** It is common sense that all physical activity burns calories. The more intense the activity, the more you burn. And as a bonus by-product, moderate to vigorous activity or exercise, particularly in the morning, will reduce your food cravings for most of the day.

- **Strong muscles:** Movement is good, but exercise is always better. If you can move through a full range of motions with some hand weights added each day—or even three to four days a week—you will not only look good with toned muscles, but you also will keep yourself flexible with strong joints, tendons, and ligaments. We are only replacing what our bodies used to do before moderation. Fifty or so years ago, before computer-controlled robots and the like, there were more jobs that required heavy lifting and constant movement. The fitness industry was very small. Now, with most jobs requiring little movement, the fitness industry is booming.

- **Blood flow:** Movement, activity, and exercise keep your blood flowing smoothly. And limiting damage to blood vessels decreases the risk of cardiovascular disease.

- **Controlling your blood sugar:** If you are already overweight, you really need to start exercising for this one. Although vigorous movement and increased activity will help, you also need to have sensible eating habits like smaller portion sizes and replacing processed foods with fresh fruit and vegetables. This is an absolute must to shed unwanted, unsightly, uncomfortable, and most important, unhealthy kilos. And it will create stable blood sugar levels to prevent the onset of a mostly lifestyle-induced condition: type 2 diabetes.

Added to these are bonuses:

- Boosting your energy with improved muscle strength

- Keeping you looking healthier with glowing skin, living longer, and looking younger

  o Exercise increases your aerobic capacity; more oxygen is moved through your body to create healthier cells. Healthier cells live longer and look better.

- Reducing stress levels and improving your mood

  o This makes for a better night of sleep.

- Boosting your immune system to fight infections, having fewer heart attacks, reducing the risk of cancer, having better organ function, and consistently living a happier and longer life

- Pumping blood to all of your body, including your brain, which should not only make you think clearly but also help with memory and learning

  o It is also responsible for releasing chemicals like endorphins to improve your mood, even though you thought you were already feeling OK. That being said, don't you think it would help reduce the risk of illnesses like dementia as well as Alzheimer's and Parkinson's diseases?

Move now to avoid future pain!

Why Any Movement is Good

Every movement that your body makes requires some part of your body to work making all movement beneficial.If you can move vigorously enough to increase your heart rate for a period of time, if you can build up some sort of aerobic fitness (aerobic fitness is measured by how good your heart and lungs are at getting oxygen into your system), and if you can do it often enough, you will start to transfer fatty deposits from the walls of your blood vessels (due to a bad lifestyle) to your muscles. These fatty deposits can be burnt off with more activity instead of the fat continually building up around your internal organs.

All humans were designed to move. I can't mention this enough: all movement is good. Just doing more than you are doing now will help you get started. Most people need to do more. There's no "one size fits all." You have to find an exercise, sport, or robust activity you like. You may find several options and mix them up. Whatever makes your heart sing, try to do something every day that makes you happy.

Gradual gain = No pain

Physical activity and sensible eating habits go hand in hand. One will complement the other. Whichever one you start first, the other one seems to follow. Getting started can be the hardest part. My next chapter on procrastination should help.

Chapter 3

Procrastination

Habitual procrastination = a life full of regrets

There is no blame and no shame in acknowledging that things need to change before an opportunity is lost. What a great first step! People will admire and envy you. You may not be a habitual procrastinator in everything you do. Most things in life may come easily to you. You may meet challenges head on and think nothing of the skill and abilities it takes to achieve. You may just get on with life. But you also may have difficulty starting a more active lifestyle or exercise program to lose weight and improve your health and quality of life. Other people who are very active may put off jobs they find challenging but that you find easy and routine. Let's call it selective procrastination.

Ask for help.

There is no shame in asking for help. In fact, recognising a problem and seeking help is a sign of strength. Find a friend to help—and a friend you can help. Find someone with the same interests who believes in you, and you can then encourage each other. In the fitness industry, they are called buddies. It is not uncommon for some self-motivated, active people to have exercise buddies. Changing what you do and starting something new can be exciting and sometimes a little scary. You may have self-doubt and think, *What if I fail?*

Exercise buddies work for each other.

I have a small gym in my converted garage. I train a few friends and a few clients on a regular basis. I charge very little per session (referred to in Aussie slang as "beer money" or "mates' rates") because, since retiring from full-time work, I have preferred to help other people as a way of giving my life purpose.

Several ladies regularly come to train three or four times a week and have been doing so for a long time. They are long past reaching their weight-loss and fitness goals. I ask them why they still keep coming. I say, "You know by now what and how to do everything. I can teach you no more." And their answer is always the same: "If I didn't have a commitment to come to train, I wouldn't do it on my own." So I began to ask myself, "Would I do as much if they did not turn up?" And the answer is, "No. I most definitely would not." So I am using them as my motivation and training buddies.

If you struggle with commitment, find a training buddy. One training buddy usually works best, as you are less likely to let one person down if you know you are leaving him or her on his or her own. If you have more buddies, it might be too easy to make an excuse to give a day a miss because you know there won't be just one person on his or her own.

Your buddy becomes invaluable whenever you experience the disappointing feeling of being inadequate. And you become invaluable to your buddy in the same way. If you are struggling, have a good laugh together and push on. You will be surprised how that struggle will turn into something easy to do, and you will soon be patting each other on the back or giving a high-five. The joy and pride you will experience when you achieve your goal will be written all over your face for all to see.

Tell someone your goals.

If you are unable to find an exercise or activity buddy, tell a close friend or family member—someone you see often—the goals you have set for yourself. This will make you more accountable. You will not want to let yourself or your confidant down because he or she cares about your health and well-being although anyone is different. A small percentage of people, including myself, will want to keep new changes or challenges in their lives secret to avoid the added pressure of friends, workout buddies, or family members asking how things are going. This type of person has to be able to inspire and motivate himself or herself.

Think of it as stopping an existing behaviour rather than starting a new one.

Just do it. And let the momentum gather.

Be assertive. Get a grip on yourself. Find the time, and do it. Do not live under the illusion that things are going to change if you don't change them. Focus your energies on accomplishing your goals. Don't think, *Can I actually do this?* Of course you can! Stepping out of your comfort zone can be exciting.

Start off with small steps—baby steps always going forward. Take the steps one at a time and achieve small goals. Then use that momentum to build on your first achievements. This way you will feel less trapped in any decision you have made or goal you have set. Once you enjoy the success and the reward of your gains, you will come to love to challenge yourself.

Set a regular time.

Schedule a set time for exercise. Most people prefer a morning session when their energy levels are high; others prefer an afternoon session after work so they can recharge. Stick to that time so you set a regular pattern that you won't want to stop or break.

Set out reminders.

Leave yourself reminder notes. The refrigerator door seems to be the most popular spot. It is usually the most-opened door or the bathroom mirror, both are hard to avoid.

Don't listen to criticism.

Do not allow others to discourage you. Pay no attention to criticism you might receive from people who are still sitting on the lounge. Do not let others tell you what you can or cannot do. They don't want you to show them up. Your progress may make them realise what a destructive lifestyle they are living, and they may not like it. Quit using excuses like, "It's all too hard, and my old life habits are too embedded." Form life-changing, sustainable habits to achieve a better life.

Do not overcomplicate things. Know what needs to be done and how to do it. No haze; all clarity.

Think about what a great feeling it would be if, after a few months of your new lifestyle, you have achieved good results that everyone can see and you are able to encourage some of those doubters—the ones still sitting on the lounge who are jealous of the new you—to join you. To me that would be the ultimate motivation to keep going and lead by example.

What if I don't?

Motivate yourself by imagining the worst-case scenario and the consequences of your inaction. If you are obese and leading a sedentary lifestyle, I won't delude you. If you don't make lifestyle changes, your body will start to deteriorate. This will greatly increase your chances of developing heart problems, type 2 diabetes, and high blood pressure. And the list goes on. Scare yourself into action! If you don't want to lose your independence and become a burden to others, act now. To turn your life around you need—I repeat—sensible eating habits, plenty of activity, a purpose in life, and very importantly, good sleep every night. The good night's sleep will fall into place and happen automatically after you adapt good eating habits, a more active lifestyle, and you give your life purpose.

Finally, if all else fails and you find you are still struggling to move out of your comfort zone, try expanding that zone by taking small steps at a time and slowly increasing your confidence to make bigger steps.

It's okay to slip occasionally; that's part of being human—as long as you get straight back up! Remember, you fail *only* if you do not get back up.

You can learn something every time you move forward again after you stumble, fail, or feel as though you have taken a step backwards. Each time you move forward will take you one step closer to your desired goal and success. It's just around the corner!

If you fail to start, there is still hope.

If you fail to start for whatever reason—temporary injury, health problems, or another reason—always keep your intent to start. The longer you leave it, the harder it will become to begin, so start as soon as possible before you lose your intent.

Before I explain some great exercise options, let's talk about good posture, which is a must. My next chapter will tell you everything you need to know.

Procrastination now = Possible pain later

Chapter 4

Posture

Achieving perfect posture 24/7.

Everything you do in life should be done where possible with correct posture: work, rest, and play!

Maintaining good posture at work.

Some of us get to move around.

Whether you are a tradesman, a builder, a plumber, an electrician, a motor mechanic, or you work in a service industry, you will be moving around most of the day, which is great. Good walking and standing posture is important. Here's a good way to remember this: "walk tall with attitude and pride." Keep your head up, your eyes focused forward, your chest out, your shoulders back. But your arms should be relaxed and slightly bent with a natural swing. Engage your core muscles by pulling your stomach in, which can give you that "standing tall" feeling. Keep your natural stride. Everyone will be different, but feet should be pointing straight ahead. Maintain a simple heel-and-toe gait with your heel striking the ground first followed by your arch and then the ball of your foot, finally pushing off again with the ball of your foot and your toes. Many people attend an occupational health and safety course at work. Possibly one of the most important messages, apart from staying safe in the workplace, is to bend your knees and keep a straight back when lifting an object from a low level.

Some of us must stand all day.

If you are required to stand most of the day, posture should be similar to those who are more active: "stand tall with attitude and pride." In management circles, this is called the "power" stance or walk.

Some of us must sit all day.

Sitting for long periods of time can have a negative impact on your body. Look for every opportunity to stand and move during the day. These breaks should include whole-body movement to restore circulation and relieve muscle tension. Breaking it down, let's start with your legs. Excess periods of sitting with little or no activity leads to weaker bones, poor circulation, muscle degeneration, and associated problems. Try standing or, if possible, taking a short walk once an hour. Apart from stretching your legs, toning your muscles, improving blood flow and bone density, an added bonus is an opportunity to be mentally refreshed. Your back (vertebral column or spine) was designed for expanding and contracting movements. Long periods of sitting can cause the vertebrae (bones or vertebral discs in the spinal column) to compress. Take every available opportunity to roll your shoulders back and open up your spine by reaching up towards the ceiling or sky. Movement, even if only for a short period, performed at regular intervals will help maintain flexibility. Let's move up to your shoulders and neck. Poor posture—leaning forward or being in a slouch position—causes aching neck and shoulders, which should be avoided where possible. This can go unnoticed. So, whether sitting, walking, or standing, as always keep your head up and shoulders back.

Correct sitting posture:

• If possible, choose a chair without armrests or remove them if possible. If they are a permanent fixture, adjust them so your elbows lift you out of a slouch position and your shoulders are square and relaxed. If there are no armrests, you will naturally tend to sit up straight and not slump in a lazy position.

• Adjust your seat height so that your feet are flat on the floor and you knees are parallel with your buttocks.

• Push your hips back as far as possible so you are sitting tall.

• If possible, adjust the back of your seat into the full upright position for full back support.

• Become a fidget at your desk: move your legs often, occasionally lift your backside off the seat. Be conscious of your posture at all times, and whenever possible, stand and move around while answering the phone.

• If it is not possible for you to stand, try pushing your seat back and lifting the lower part of your legs up.

• Stretch while seated at your desk—in any and all directions. Reach for the sky, try to touch your toes, reach forward, backwards, and sideways.

Conduct a basic postural assessment.

Here is a basic static postural assessment that you can do yourself at home. It is quick, easy to understand, and very important. It is taken from my first book, and is certainly worth a review.

Stand in your bare feet with your back against a wall (no skirting board if possible). Head, buttocks, and heels should all touch the wall, and your feet should point straight out. You should feel your body weight in your heels and not have that feeling of falling forward. Check the space between the wall and your lower back by sliding your hand, in a flat position, into the space. If your knuckles fit snugly between your lower back and the wall, the arch of your is acceptable. However, if you can pass a closed fist between the space, you will probably need professional help.

In the same position, check your shoulders. If the middle of your upper back touches the wall but your shoulders round forward away from the wall, you need to work on exercising your upper back muscles to pull them back. You also would benefit from stretching the chest muscles.

Remember, this is a very quick assessment designed to get you thinking and to motivate you to work for a healthier lifestyle. If you have any concerns, please consult your health care professional.

Maintaining good posture while at rest.

Posture while you sleep.

"What's he on about now?" you may ask. "Don't we ever get a break?" Considering that we spend one-third of our life in bed, it is worthwhile giving good posture during sleep a try, unless you have sleep apnoea or a medical condition which may prevent you from trying different positions while lying in bed.

You should first start with a great mattress and a firm to medium-firm, good-quality pillow, both of which should give you good support. We want to keep your neck in its natural curved position, and a very soft pillow or multiple pillows will not do that.

Sleeping flat on your back with legs straight and arms by your side is the best position for your neck and spine. You may look like you have passed away, but it is still the best position. Sleeping on your left side with your legs bent in a comfortable and natural position will aid circulation and heart function. As we will normally change position several times each night, you will get the best of both worlds. Avoid sleeping on your stomach, as this prevents you from keeping a neutral spine position, which will result in back, neck, and joint problems.

As we all have a twenty-four-hour body clock, which is built in and regulates our daily cycle, keeping consistent sleep patterns is important. When possible, try to get a good eight hours of sleep every night at roughly the same time. As far as possible, unless you are sick, try not to overextend your sleep hours on your days off or on weekends, inviting as it may be. I am not talking an hour or two, or having a relaxed reading of the newspaper with a cuppa; I am referring to a long sleep until late morning, as this can result in a feeling similar to minor jet lag. Anyone, including myself, who has worked a night shift will know the feeling I am referring to. If you are a regular shift worker, I do not know the answer except, as we do when getting over jet lag, try to resume regular normal sleeping hours as soon as possible.

Everybody is different and has different requirements; this is general advice.

Maintaining good posture at play.

Pay attention to posture during all activities.

Having good posture while at play or exercising is more important than at any other time because your body is usually under more stress. Try to keep your body in alignment at all times. When standing, try to imagine a straight vertical line from your ears to your ankles. This should align your shoulders, trunk, thighs, and knees. This alignment method is true for most exercise. "The plank" position is a great example: your legs, back, and your neck should resemble a straight line with no sagging or "popping up" in the trunk. And elbows should be straight under your shoulders, forming ninety-degree angles at your shoulders, chest, and elbows. Any deviation from this alignment can potentially set you up for injury by causing more pressure on your joints. This may not be true for every movement, but it is a good guide. When performing the plank, which I think is one of the best exercises you can do, the most common mistake people make is placing their elbows in front of their shoulders and allowing their heads to sag. Your head should be up, and you should be looking at a spot just in front of your hands. This will avoid any strain on your neck muscles.

As a reminder, here are the plank instructions from my previous book: Start off on the floor on your hands and knees. Engage your core muscles to support your body weight and lower yourself down so you are resting the front part of your body on your elbows and forearms. Holding your hands together, extend one leg back so it is resting on its toes. Do the same with the other leg. You whole body is now supported on your toes, elbows, and forearms. Correct posture is head up, looking at a spot just in front of your hands. Your shoulders to your ankles must resemble a plank (it should be as flat as a board). Keeping those core muscles engaged, hold the position for as long as you can. Do not expect to stay "up" for too long. Even ten seconds is a good start. If you are overweight or not yet very strong, try extending one leg at a time until you become stronger.

Pay attention to posture while driving.

Some of us spend many hours every day driving a car, so it is important to be conscious of our posture for that period of time. Next time you get behind the steering wheel, turn the ignition to the on position without starting the car, the dashboard will light up like a Christmas tree, and your car computer will check that all systems are go. It's time for you to check your driving posture.

Sit in the seat so you are square with the steering wheel. Adjust the back of the seat as you would your desk chair, with a slight backwards recline. Align your back so you have equal support or pressure covering the whole length of your back from your buttocks to your shoulders, as if you are squeezed into your seat. Adjust the seat distance so that, when you have the brake pedal fully depressed, your knees remain slightly bent or "soft." If your knees are straight, you are too far back. If your knees are at a ninety-degree angle, you are too close. Use the same guide for your arms, keeping your elbows soft. Head up, shoulders back, and off you go. Remember to keep that good posture for the entire length of your journey. Don't crumple or slump in the seat. Keep your spine in its natural *S* shape rather than a hunched-over *C* shape.

Good posture now = No back pain later

Now that you have achieved good posture—and it has cost you nothing—let's look at your exercise time as quality time.

Chapter 5

Maximising the Benefits
of Your Exercise Time

Your exercise or gym time can be precious time squeezed into a busy day, so let us use that time to the best advantage possible. Most people are satisfied during the gym, training, or exercise session with repetitive, boring exercise, which I have no doubt is great for your body; but we could benefit further.

All the hard work so many people do in the gym is to reduce weight, obtain a better fitness level, and achieve a great, toned body. I have no problem with that at all, but why stop there? I think we can achieve much more. I suggest we can improve our coordination and balance, and reduce the chance—or forestall the onset—of mental impairment greatly, simply by challenging our brain as we exercise. Why spend endless hours on a mindless, tedious apparatus like a treadmill listening to music to break the boredom? I do, however, believe "cardio" machines can be great for warming up or for short periods during in a circuit training session. Why not make your gym exercise and sports training of all types more exciting, challenging, and beneficial?

Let's improve our coordination.

Balancing your brain and improving your coordination is as simple as using your non-dominant hand more often, this being the hand you would not normally throw a ball with or write with.

Start by doing simple tasks at first to avoid causing any damage. If your dominant hand is your right hand, try opening a door or brushing your teeth with your left hand. Gradually move on to more difficult tasks. Using your non-dominant hand is difficult and forces you to intensify your concentration as you direct your thoughts and focus on areas you would not normally focus on. This will exercise your brain. As it is any time you begin something new, you must give yourself time to master the challenge and develop a better and more harmonious balance combination between your right and left sides. In the gym, most exercises are balanced, so try picking up a light medicine ball (move to a heavier ball once you become proficient) and throwing it to a partner or against a solid wall and catching it on return with your non-dominant hand. You can kick a ball around a local park with your non-dominant foot.

I cannot think of a sporting challenge that would not benefit from improved balance, coordination, and an alert brain.

Let's improve our balance.

How do we work on improving our balance? Simple—all exercise is good, but we should put some extra time into our core area—the muscles front and back between and under your shoulders and down to your lower waist or hip area. That is your centre of gravity. Combine this exercise with good posture to greatly reduce the chances of accidental falls. The importance of preventing falls increases significantly as we age.

A great static balance test is to stand on one leg with the other leg raised to form a simple right angle at the knee. Raise the opposite arm straight out and hold a light weight. Keep this position for ten seconds then close your eyes and see how long you last. Most people last only a few seconds, so keep practicing. This posture will improve your balance. Use it to put some fun into an exercise break.

A great exercise to improve confidence in your balance is to practice, practice, practice a stationary lunge. When you feel comfortable with the stationary lunge, move onto a walking lunge.

To correctly perform a lunge, start by assuming a good standing posture. Take a step forward then drop your body straight down. Compare this to showing reverence in a church: "genuflect." If you need support to keep your balance, place one hand on the back of a chair. Gradually remove your hand, but leave the chair there for security. As your confidence grows, remove the chair altogether. Your rear knee should almost reach the ground, and both legs should form a right angle at the knees. Keep your head up and your back straight. Push back up to complete one repetition (rep). Correct technique is straight up and straight down; do not lean forward.

For a stationary (or static) lunge, repeat each lunge on the same spot. For a walking lunge, take a step forward with each lunge.

To compound the exercise and to test and improve your balance, try reaching down and touching your forward foot with either hand as you step forward.

I always say that we do core exercises to prevent having a fall, and we do strength training and weight-resistant exercises, which help with our bone density, just in case we do have a fall. Our bone mass reaches its peak at a younger age than you may think. It is not in your forties or fifties; rather, it is in our thirties. And as our bones react positively to resistance or weight-bearing exercise, everyone who can possibly exercise should do so even if it is a only for a short period of time on most days of the week. Doing things today that you may not feel like doing will help you do things in later life that others who have led a sedentary, inactive lifestyle will not be able to do.

Your body was designed for movement and work, so to keep it strong and flexible. Use it now, and use it often.

No one wants mental impairment.

More and more, the common opinion from medical research and trials is that exercise decreases the risk of suffering from dementia or any other mental impairment, so keep your exercise session exciting and your mind active. The way to do this is to add plenty of variety and aerobic fun exercises to every session, exercise which will keep you thinking of your next move. Don't forget to test yourself by taking every opportunity to challenge your brain by using your non-dominant hand; this will keep you sharp and reduce your risk of dementia. Practising mindfulness while you exercise will improve your mood whilst having a profoundly positive impact on anxiety. This will lead to improved self-esteem, which must put your brain in a good place.

When you are physically strong, you will feel emotionally strong, and vice versa. The stronger you get with exercise, the stronger mentally you will become, and when you are faced with adversity, you will be able to remain composed and in control.

Exercise is often considered to be the opposite of relaxation or sleeping, but they do have a common theme—both exercise and rest give you time to clear your head and give you that feeling of being connected with your body.

Healthy brain = No pain

If you are new to exercise, then you are one of the people I am trying to reach. High-intensity interval training may be new to you, but no longer needs to be. Read on.

Chapter 6

My Version of High-Intensity Interval Training

High-intensity interval training (HIIT) is the best way to train for weight loss and fitness.

Intense exercise efforts are interspersed with rest periods. Anyone who has been a regular gym user or has been involved with active sport requiring a medium to high level of fitness will have heard of high-intensity interval training. This book is designed for people who are not already converted to the huge benefits of a regular exercise regime. Interval training is a relatively recent training method, replacing the old, steady route—long-period training sessions; for example, taking a long jog round and round an oval.

I think HIIT is a great way to train. It can be adapted to almost any form of exercise because it simply involves varying the intensity level, although I believe the experts leave out the most important word. I call it high-intensity *short*-interval training. You can also add the words *active rest* after *interval* so it becomes **high-intensity short-interval active-rest training (HISIART)**—a long name, but a great way to train to get great results.

Let's break it down into stages.

High intensity:

You are going to go as hard as you can at a suitable exercise and for as long as you can—running on the spot, riding an exercise bike, or doing jumping jacks. The object is just to get your heart rate up as quickly as possible.

Short intervals:

You may maintain this high intensity for thirty to sixty seconds, depending on your fitness level.

Active rest:

You can also refer to this period as active recovery. This is the period to bring your heart rate back down. Walk around, move your arms in every direction, or perform any low-intensity movement. The goal is to rest while still being active. Remember to take plenty of deep breaths. The time period for active rest will vary depending on fitness level, difficulty of exercise, time duration, and so forth. To me, the time period you spend in active rest is not as important as how hard you go in the high-intensity section, and that you must return to high-intensity activity as soon as your heart rate drops. It is all about causing the heart rate to go up and down, and repeating the cycle.

This form of training has many advantages.

If you are overweight and looking to burn calories to reduce fat, it seems to be an accepted fact that HISIART is more effective in accelerating fat loss than the steady running-around-the-oval method (or using a cardio machine at a steady pace). The more intense you make the exercise, the more oxygen your body consumes, and this can create an after-burn effect. Your metabolism can remain increased for twenty-four to forty-eight hours with interval training.

If running is for you and you have a park to use, I find the grass surface to be a little kinder on your joints than a concrete path or asphalt road—and a lot safer. Our bodies were designed to run barefoot in soft soil. Adapt to interval training by simply adding a few sprints to bring your heart rate up and a light jog as your active rest to reduce your heart rate.

Here are some of the many advantages of HISIART:

- You certainly will not get bored, and it can be fun.

- Most people will feel more energised. A longer period of training at a moderate rate can make you feel drained.

- It takes less time to get a better result.

- You will enter the fat-burning zone faster.

- The new muscles you develop can assist in burning body fat even while you rest.

- More oxygen is consumed during training, which means your body will still burn fat after training.

- Some people believe (and I support the fact) that HISIART improves brain function.

- With no heavy weights involved, HISIART is suitable for a wide range of people and can be carried out in a small or large area, indoors or outside.

There are a few things to be aware of.

I have mentioned that, with HISIART, you will enter the fat-burning zone faster, but you will also enter muscular-breakdown zone faster. Preventing injury should always be the first priority. Keep it simple to start. Your body will be shocked and pushed to its limits. Pain is an indication that you may be doing damage to your muscles. Progress in a slow manner; if you push beyond the pain boundaries, you may experience a slow recovery time.

This may seem like a contradiction: you are asked to push as hard as you can for a short period, but not so hard that you risk injury. This is correct. You are the best judge. No pain is necessary to get results; all movement is good. If you can handle a small amount of muscle burn, that is all that is required to keep you moving forward. You will find as you progress that the length of time you spend in high-intensity activity before you experience muscle burn will increase. The exercise will become easier and more enjoyable.

If high-intensity training terrifies you because you are uncoordinated, overweight, or just new to exercise, just adapt slowly. Build on what you do have, and ease into HISIART. Go for a walk, and increase the intensity and length little by little. Almost any body size and ability can benefit from this form of exercise. Remember, you are the best judge of how you feel. You know best when your heart rate is up, your muscles are starting to burn, and you are feeling fatigued. You control the interval—both the intensity and the length. And you return after active rest only when your heart rate is back to almost normal. I say almost because it is a training session; you are working hard, and you should expect your heart rate to be above rest level most of the time.

Here's a great HISIART routine:

This is one of my favourite forms of high-intensity training. It provides a very low risk of injury and is easy on your joints, but is guaranteed to set your metabolism on fire and keep burning fat for hours after your training session has finished.

You will need a stationary bike and a clock with a second hand. First, warm up on the bike and select a resistance level or program that is a little difficult. Position the clock so you can easily see it, or have a buddy time you. Some exercise bikes have a time readout you can use to count the seconds. To begin, go as fast as you can on the bike for eight seconds then ease off. Do not stop; rather, keep pedalling at a slower rate for twelve seconds. So, this is eight seconds of high intensity and twelve seconds of active rest. Three repetitions equal one minute, which makes the time periods easy to keep track off. Start with four- or five-minute sessions, or continue until your leg muscles become a little uncomfortable. Slowly increase the session time and resistance level, giving your body time to adjust and build muscle strength to avoid muscle fatigue and pain.

Once you can do eight to ten minutes without feeling too much distress, add the exercise to a balanced exercise program three to four times a week. This would be a perfect addition to either or both of the exercise formats I describe in the next chapters—boxing and kettlebells.

Up next: my two favourite exercise formats.

My next two chapters will provide all the information you need about what I believe are the best two forms of exercise formats: boxing and kettlebells.

By regularly using my version of both formats you can achieve fantastic results:

> Ladies, you will not only achieve great overall muscle tone, you will still remain feminine with sexy legs, a tight and cheeky butt, and firm perky bust line.

> Men, you will achieve a lean, sportsman look with toned, natural-looking muscles.

There is no need to feel intimidated by either format. I will fully explain both. They are designed to keep you interested with low-impact fun moves. I have also taken into account the fact that most people's bodies are motivated to avoid pain and to seek pleasure.

Chapter 7

Boxing Format

Boxing is one of my favourite forms of exercise. I am not talking about training yourself so you can knock an opponent senseless. I'm not talking about making the exercise too complex. It's more about adapting the boxing format to a safe exercise program and turning a gym session into a fun session. Boxing will take you away from the boring treadmill and weight machines.

I have designed a program that is not as physically and mentally demanding as, say, a boot camp session (although it could be easily adapted to be just as difficult). Still, you will still be constantly challenged with a mixed variety of moves. You can have a high-intensity, short-interval, active-rest training session that will tone your entire body. Plus, the low-impact moves are easy on your joints. By adding exercise moves, you will be incorporating large muscle groups together, compounding every move for maximum benefit.

Boxing suits all age groups as well as body sizes and shapes. I know of many petite mature-age ladies who just love it. Boxing is not about building big muscles; it will not bulk you up. It will make you feel trim, taut, and terrific.

Boxercise is fun and provides multiple benefits!

I do not know of any other particular exercise format that can provide all the following benefits:

- Requires a high level of mental focus

- Builds hand-eye coordination

- Improves balance and body coordination because, by throwing a punch, we are exerting a force away from our centre of gravity

- Offers an opportunity to easily vary the intensity

- Improves reaction time (speed) and agility (light in movement)

- Builds muscular endurance and strength

- Increases cardio fitness

- Aids in weight loss

- Tones most, if not all, major muscle groups

- Improves skills and techniques that can be beneficial when applied to a large range of other sports: speed, balance, and endurance

- Releases stress, builds confidence, makes an exercise session fun

- Improves bone density

- Is certainly, without a doubt, a mood changer for the better, setting you up for the whole day

Here's how boxercize works.

These routines are all designed for two people, the boxer and focus pad holder. They can also be easily adapted to be used by one person and a hanging or freestanding punching bag. To avoid injuries and keep routines running smoothly, there can be only one boss, and that is the person holding the focus pad. He or she calls all the shots and must have complete control. This will minimise the mistakes and maximise the fun and benefits gained.

Remember, you each get a turn as pad holder. I suggest you change over frequently to even out the load on the boxer. Only one type of punch is thrown, and I will describe it in a bit. This keeps the exercise simple, less demanding, and more appealing to all kinds of people. Hopefully it will also keep the exercise accident free. To perfect the correct technique for other punches like uppercuts, hooks, and so forth would be physically demanding, take up too much time, and distract you from the exercise component. All the exercises intertwined with a basic boxing moves are designed to hold your interest, get you fit, and achieve a great, toned body.

Let's find a partner and get our equipment together:

You do not need a lot of equipment, so I suggest you make it top-of-the-range. Quality leather never seems to wear. I use my gloves and pads five days a week, and they are still in good condition after five years.

You can work with a training buddy or a hanging or freestanding punching bag. You, or you and your buddy, will need the following additional equipment:

- One pair of good-quality leather boxing gloves. The wrist area should be wide and thick with a Velcro strap so it can be easily tightened if needed to avoid wrist sprain. The knuckle region should be well padded and pre-curved. The thumb should be attached by elastic to the main glove area; to avoid injury, you do not want your thumb sticking out.

- A good-quality focus pad with sufficient padding to absorb the constant impact as it catches punches. A curved pad is important because it is better at absorbing the impact from a curved glove.

- Two or more pairs of cotton inner gloves (for each of you if you work with a buddy) that can be washed frequently and reused. The cotton gloves prevent your leather gloves from developing an odour, particularly if you train in a warm climate. The cotton gloves also prevent the transfer of germs when you swap gloves and focus pads with your buddy.

Here are some rules for fun boxercise:

Follow these rules for a fun, enjoyable, safe, injury-free, and beneficial session:

- Do not make your combination and routine too complex; keep it simple, and keep it safe.

- Always perform your moves in slow motion first and take time to learn your routine using good posture and technique before you add speed.

- Men, you do not have to punch hard to gain benefit. You only increase the risk of injury to yourself or your training buddy. It's all about posture, technique, speed, agility, and endurance.

I will mention this early and I will mention this often because it caused the only injury I have ever suffered in a training session, and I am seventy-two, l and have been exercising all my adult life: *When using the focus pad, keep your elbows tucked in close to your body.*

Now, we'll move on to technique.

Techniques for the focus pad holder:

Let's start with the most important person, the focus pad holder. The person boxing has all the fun; the focus pad holder, who may not exert as much energy, has all the responsibility. You cannot stand there and hold the pad up in just any position. This job requires a lot of concentration, skill, good posture, and correct technique. But the technique is easy, fun to learn, and can be quickly mastered. The pad holder provides resistance to the boxer's punches, neutralising part of the impact and constantly absorbing some of the impact force of each punch. Following these techniques holds true when using one or two focus pads.

The person holding the focus pad controls all the moves in the training session and is the boss. Follow these techniques:

- Assume good standing posture: a split stance with one foot a step behind the other. This will give you the best possible balance, and with balance comes control.

- Hold the pad up so that the top of the pad is roughly at the height of the boxer's eyes, so you can move forward and down to the boxers punch, neutralising some of the force.

- Keep your elbows in. Do not hold your elbows outside of your body/ shoulder line. This will prevent shoulder injury. Keep your forearms upright from your elbow and close to your biceps (upper front arm muscle) so you can naturally move quickly and downwards onto the boxer's punch.

- As the boxer punches, move the pad forward into the punch. The gloves should hit the pad when they are approximately half way through the punch. There will be a bouncing effect. Do not keep pushing forward; instead, flick back to absorb some of the impact. This prevents wrist and shoulder injury to both boxer and pad holder.

Techniques for the boxer:

The techniques I explain here are designed to integrate exercise into a boxing format and may vary greatly from pure boxing techniques. In fact, they have nothing to do with "ring craft."

I try to keep it simple, fun, and injury free. Here's how to do the punching exercise:

1. With good standing posture and a normal stance with your feet at least shoulder width apart and knees slightly bent, remain light on your feet and ready to move. You can bounce on your feet if you wish, adding to the energy you use. This stance is more akin to a martial arts movement because you are ready to move quickly in

any direction. If you are doing a prolonged punching routine of five or more punches without movement, a split stance will be highly advantageous to maintaining good balance.

2. Make sure your fingers are tightly clenched inside the good-quality boxing gloves. Keep your thumb in and make a fist like a rock.

3. I prefer to have my arm lower than a boxer in the ring would, as there is no need to protect my head from an opponent who is intent on knocking me out. Place your fists in a horizontal position and elbows kept low at a forty-five degree or right angle.

4. As you raise your arm toward the focus pad, twist your forearm and wrist so they are aligned. Your glove is now in a horizontal position with your palm facing down. Try to hit with your centre knuckles. The punch is similar to a jab only it carries a lot more movement. It is important to practice slowly until you get it right, because it all centres on how your punch hits the focus pad. Remember: tight fist, knuckles hitting flat, and wrist aligned with your forearm throughout the execution of your punch.

5. Start throwing punches towards the focus pad slowly: left, right, left, right with no particular dominant hand, as we are looking for complete balance, coordination, and good technique. I try to think of it as a "twist and pop"—you twist your arm and wrist coming forward and pop the punch as it meets the focus pad. Practice until it becomes second nature, until you can perform a good-quality punch without thinking about it, because you won't be able to think very much when you become fatigued.

It is important to maintain good form. When a punch is poorly executed and repeated time and time again, muscle damage can occur even if you don't experience any obvious signs or feel any pain.

Speed is great, but power is not of great importance to me. Trying to punch as hard as you can is of no benefit to you or your pad holder. To increase power you have to alter your stance so you can transfer weight, and this quite often can put you off balance, which causes technique to go out the window. Additionally, the pad holder can be put off balance, which is an injury risk for both of you.

Here are my custom-designed boxing routines:

First, read these tips:

As I have mentioned, these routines are all designed for two people, the boxer and focus pad holder. They can also be easily adapted to be used by one person and a punching bag.

Remember these points, which apply to all the routines:

- Always do a slow run through at the start of each routine to avoid any misunderstanding between the boxer and pad holder. Misunderstandings can lead to mishaps and injuries.

- The optimal distance between boxer and pad holder will come naturally and will vary greatly among partners, depending on the arm reach of the boxer.

- Mild muscle burn is okay, but don't continue if any pain occurs.

- Increase your heart rate without going to a point that causes your speech to be affected. Slurred speech is a great indicator of a person's state of fatique. The more fatigued you are, the more mistakes you make, and the longer it takes for you to recover.

- Maintain good posture at all times.

- The pad holder's instructions must be clear and precise; examples are: start, stop, five reps to go.

- The most common boxing injury, even when using top-notch equipment, is to the wrist and is almost always caused by poor technique repeated time and time again. At the first sign of any discomfort, stop your workouts and rest for a week. Practice again without hitting a focus pad or bag until you are proficient, which should not take long. You might just need a bit of concentration until you achieve more consistency. Then try again with a partner. Unless you are feeling frail or have a weakness caused by a previous injury, there should not be any problems.

- Keep your routines short and your breaks short to maximise benefits and fun.

Have fun with these eight boxercize routines:

Box and run:

Stand face to face with the pad holder holding the pad up, face out, elbows in and at approximately the boxer's eye level. The boxer then performs ten alternating punches, moves or slowly runs backwards for eight to ten steps, and then returns forward to the pad holder, pushing off hard and fast. That is 1 rep. Complete this routine as many times as it takes to increase your heart rate and experience some mild fatigue.

Main muscle groups used: arms, legs (front and back), core (core muscles are more engaged when running backwards).

Pad holder's job: Observe the boxer's punching technique. You will be able to feel a well-delivered punch through your focus pads. It will be flat and even with a crisp sound. Encourage the boxer and ensure his or her safety, because he or she will be running backwards, and you will have a clear view of any obstacles. Also observe the boxer for extreme fatigue. Ask the boxer to stop or slow down if his or her response is laboured or difficult to understand when you ask how he or she is doing.

Boxer's job: Concentrate on posture and technique and have fun!

Benefits gained beyond the general benefits of boxing:

- The boxer will improve muscular balance by running backwards, which builds muscles you may not normally work.

- It is a proven fact you burn more calories when walking or running backwards.

- The exercise improves posture because you will naturally keep a straight back when running backwards.

- Running backwards puts less pressure on your knees.

- Any backward movement will certainly heighten your senses and your peripheral vision.

There is a good reason I put this routine first: it is simple to perform, and so much can be achieved in a short period of time.

Boxing rounds.

This is boxing without any extra exercise added.

Pad holder's job: Move backwards, sideways, and in any direction you like in a random pattern. Vary the height from high (eye level) to low (shoulder level). Remember to keep your elbows in close to your body.

Boxer's job: Simply follow the pad, striking it with good-quality punches. Because the routine requires constant movement in various directions do not let good posture and technique go out the window.

Boxing kicks:

There is nothing about boxing in this routine. It is the only time the pad holder may hold his or her elbows away from the body.

Main muscle groups used: Leg and abdominals.

Pad holder's job: Stand at right angles to the boxer with the pad extended in front of you. Ask the boxer to kick the pads. Vary the height, starting off low and slowly moving up through a range of ten kicks on each leg.

Boxer's job: Your foot contact with the focus pad should be with the top or instep of the foot with toes flat to avoid toe damage. Take one good step backwards with the kicking leg before the kick to maximise the range of movement.

Tip: Boxer—The higher you kick the more your abdominal muscles are worked.

Benefits gained beyond the general benefits of boxing: Boxer—Good leg coordination and balance.

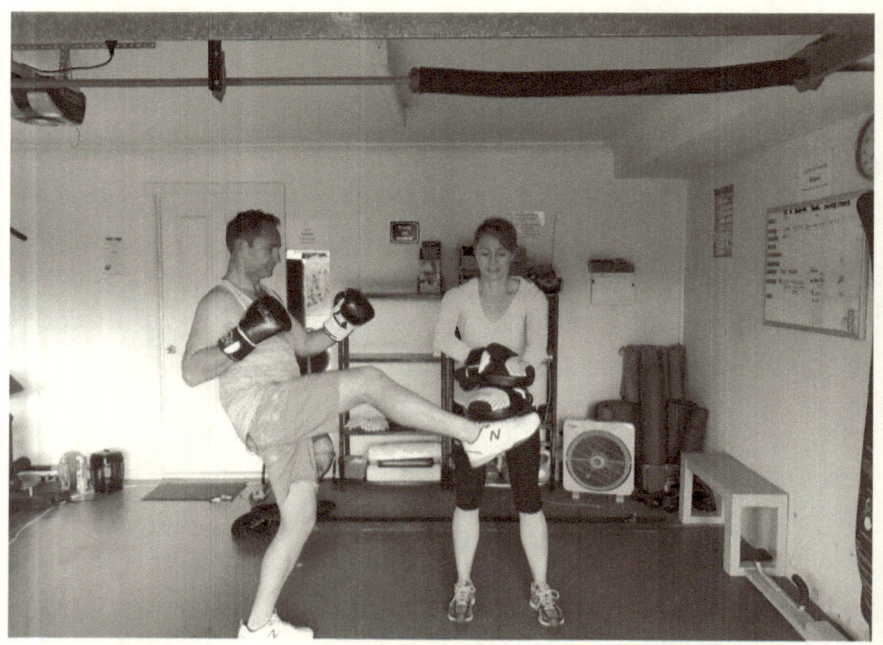

Balance kicks:

Main muscle groups used: Legs, lower back, and lower abdominals.

Pad holder's job: Stand at right angles to the boxer with the pad extended in front of you. Ask the boxer to kick the pads.

Boxer's job: Stand with one leg raised forming a right angle at the knee, arms extended at shoulder height (to help with balance). Attempt to perform ten short kicks to the pad without letting the kicking foot touch the floor.

Tip: Boxer—This is not easy. You will get better with practice.

Benefits gained beyond the general benefits of boxing: Boxer—Great for balance and to raise confidence as you improve your ability.

Boxing squats:

Main muscle groups used: Arms and legs.

Pad holder's job: Stand facing the boxer with the pad directly in front of you.

Boxer's job: Face the pad holder and deliver three punches: two in a row with the non-dominant hand and then one with the dominant hand. The theory behind this is that you are setting your opponent up for a knockout punch, but you fail and you have to take evasive action. A boxer in the ring would duck. A replacement exercise is a squat, so if you are right handed, the sequence for one rep is two left, one right then squat.

Tip: Boxer—Perform a good squat not a hunched over duck. Stay long through your spine, keep heel contact and head up. To add to the exercise and improve coordination, raise your gloves to protect your head as a boxer would.

Benefits gained beyond the general benefits of boxing: Boxer—Great legs and butt, improved co-ordination.

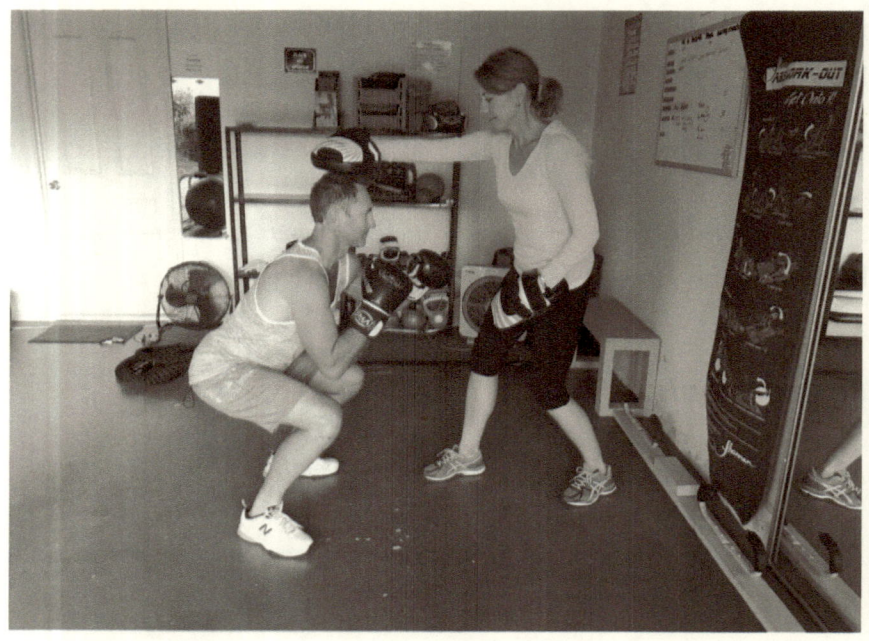

Boxing sidestep:

Main muscle groups used: Adductors (inside thigh).

Pad holder's job: Stand facing the boxer with the pad directly in front of you.

Boxer's job: Throw five alternating punches. Move five side steps to the right. Return to the pad holder. Deliver another five alternating punches. Move five side steps to the left. Repeat this as many times as you can for your fitness level.

Tip: Boxer—Maintain good posture with side steps. Keep your gloves up high.

Benefits gained beyond the general benefits of boxing: Coordination. How often do you normally move sideways?

Boxing knees up:

Main muscle groups used: Arms and legs.

Pad holder's job: Stand facing the boxer with the pad directly in front of you. Hold the pad high for the boxer's three punches and lower it for the boxer's "knee kicks."

Boxer's job: Throw three alternating punches: right, left, right. As the pad holder drops the pad, lift your right knee and "knee kick" the pad. With both feet on the floor again, repeat the same sequence, using the same knee: punch right, left, right, and then knee up. Do ten reps with each knee.

Tips: Boxer and pad holder—Concentration is a must. That upcoming knee could cause damage. Maintain the same boxing routine to avoid confusion between partners.

Benefits gained beyond the general benefits of boxing: Boxer and pad holder—Good coordination.

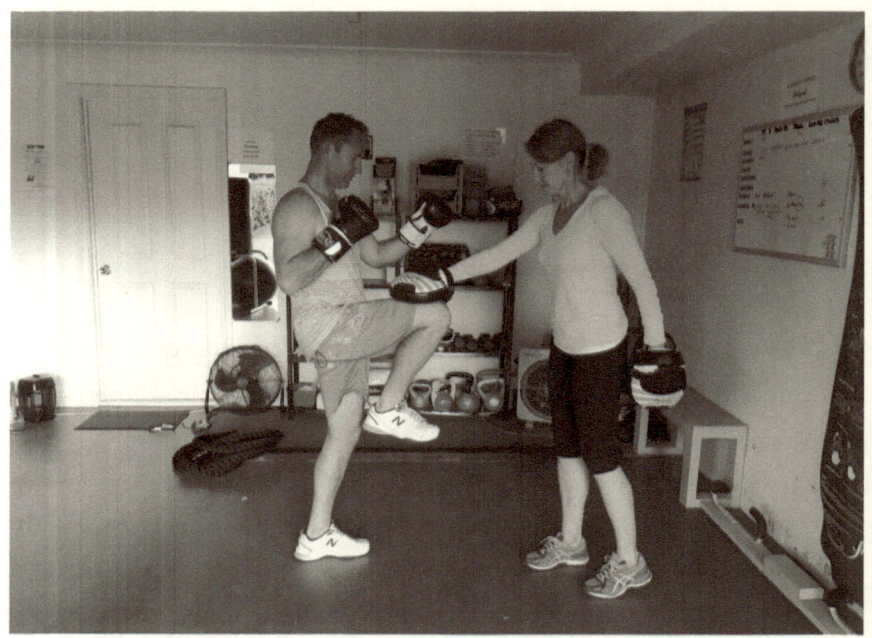

Boxing sit-up:

Main muscle groups used: Arms, legs, and abdominals.

Pad holder's job and boxer's job: Sit on a mat facing each other with your legs intertwined. Pad holder, hold the pad in front of you. Boxer, hold your gloves in front of you. Both rock back to a forty-five-degree angle and then come up to a sitting position. Boxer, deliver five alternate punches. Both return to the forty-five-degree angle position. Repeat this as many times as possible, or do five reps, have a short rest, and do five more reps. Continue until one person forfeits.

Tip: I train people to rock back to only a forty-five-degree angle between sit-ups rather than going completely to the floor position. Dead lifting from a floor position over a long period of time can cause neck problems, and I have changed my mind regarding boxing sit-up technique as well as normal sit-up technique after observing people over many years.

Benefits gained beyond the general benefits of boxing: This exercise works more muscle areas in one exercise than you would normally do, plus you get to learn how coordinated your partner is.

I have designed all of these boxing exercise routines for weight loss, fitness, muscle toning, improved coordination, and body-and-mind balance. They can easily be adapted into a great HISIART session simply by increasing the intensity (speed of movement) and using more frequent but shorter rest breaks. You can even add additional exercises like push-ups, and you can pyramid your exercise. Here's an example: five punches followed by ten push-ups, and then five more punches and nine push-ups, and so on until you reach one push-up. Then you move back down the pyramid until you complete ten push-ups again. Or you can vary the intensity to a more leisurely pace. If you make a mistake, have a laugh and carry on. All movement is good. There is no need for pain.

Incredible gain and no pain.

Chapter 8

Kettlebells Explained

A kettlebell is simply a sphere-shaped weight with a handle, and you need only one. It is small, portable, and comes with its own convenient carry handle. You can use it almost anywhere, anytime, and you need only a small space to do the exercises—in a room in your home or out in the park on a nice day.

If you are looking for weight loss, fitness, and a great body shape, whatever the boxing format may miss (which would be very little) the kettlebell routine will more than cover, add to, and complement.

Here's some basic information about kettlebells.

Because the movements are simple, practical and easily performed by most people, you won't need a trainer. The fundamental movement patterns are based on everyday life movements. You can start anytime even if you are out of shape. You will start to work your body as one unit, with a whole body functional training session, combining strength training and cardio fitness. This effectively provides an overall fitness regime for practically the entire body. These non-impact exercises will not be only easy on your joints; they will strengthen your tendons and ligaments, making them less susceptible to injuries and pain.

You will not build big, bulky muscles; rather, you will build great toned muscles. Many of the exercise patterns are unique and require a wide and varied range of motion. Some moves are off centre and all of them almost always require more than one single joint movement. That means that most of my routines are compound routines that work more than one muscle area in each move. You will be quite often engaging your core muscles, including your back muscles. You are more likely to stick with your kettlebells because they are inexpensive, the exercises are quick and not boring, and best of all, your workout will deliver great results including stability, mobility, strength, cardio fitness, and mental focus.

Have fun with these six kettlebell routines.

Each of my kettlebell routines consists of a set of three moves: two standard moves that are repeated (and some are combined), and a third exercise component, which changes. The standard move takes approximately thirty seconds to complete. There are ten reps of each exercise component.

Here are the two basic standard moves you will use:

Standard move one: Around and around

Stand upright with good posture. With arms straight, swing the kettlebell around your body, switching from one hand to the other when the ball is in front of you and when it is in back of you. Do a number of reps and then change direction.

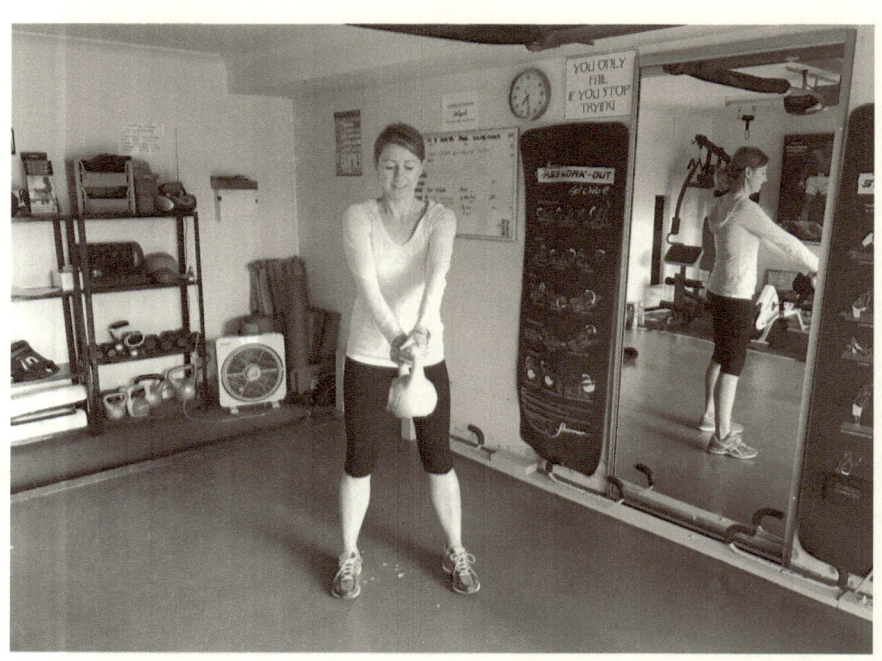

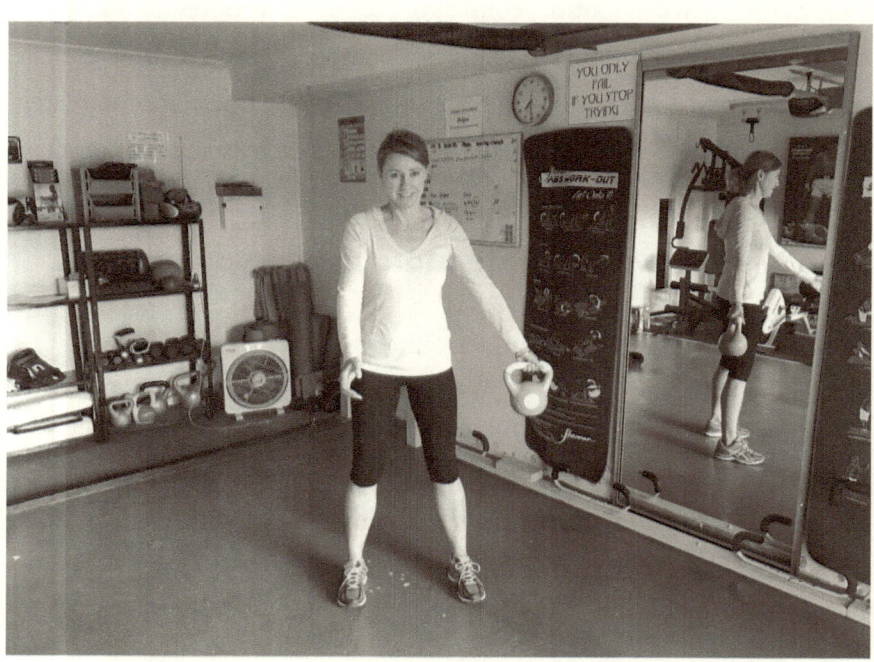

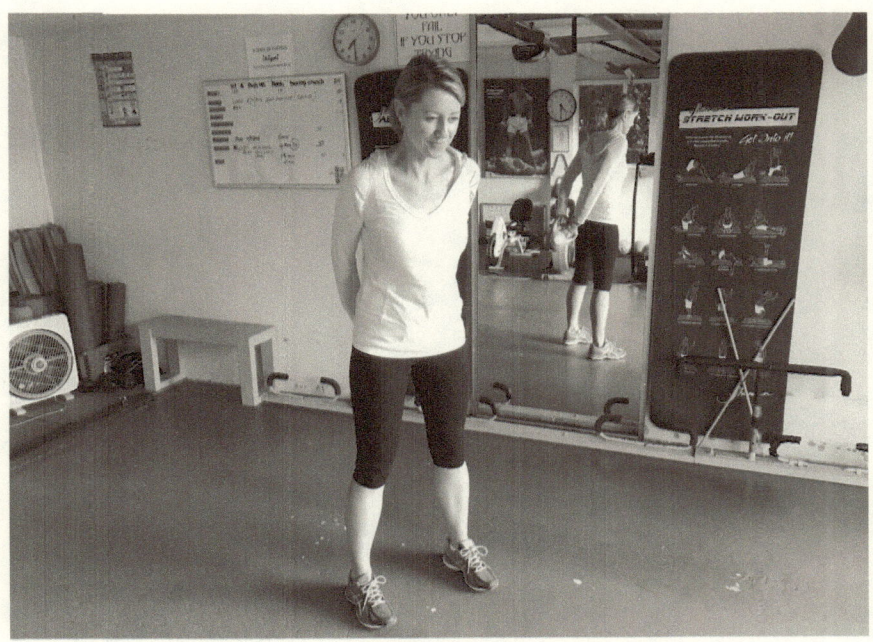

Standard move two: Figure eight

Bend at the waist and hold your back straight. Transferring the kettlebell from one hand to the other, pass the kettlebell around and between both legs in a figure eight pattern: in front of your right knee and behind your right knee with your right hand. Transfer to your left hand when the kettlebell is between your legs, and then bring it in front of your left knee and around the back of your left knee with your left hand—on and on!

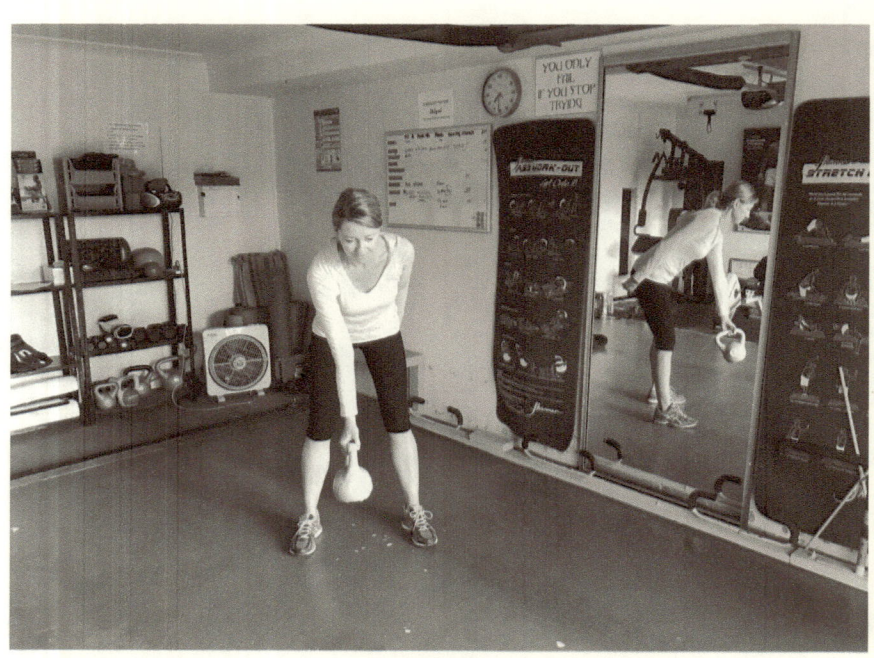

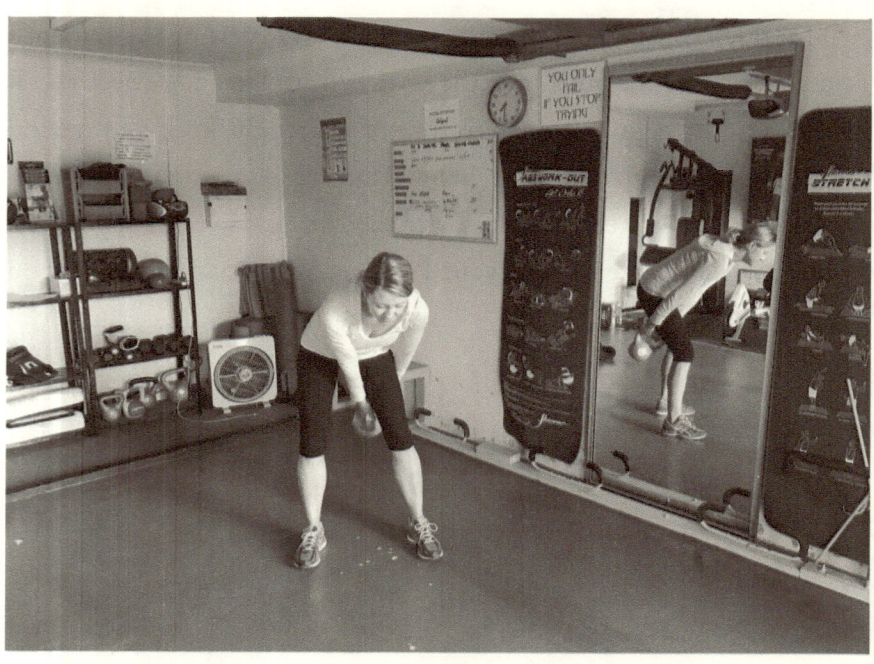

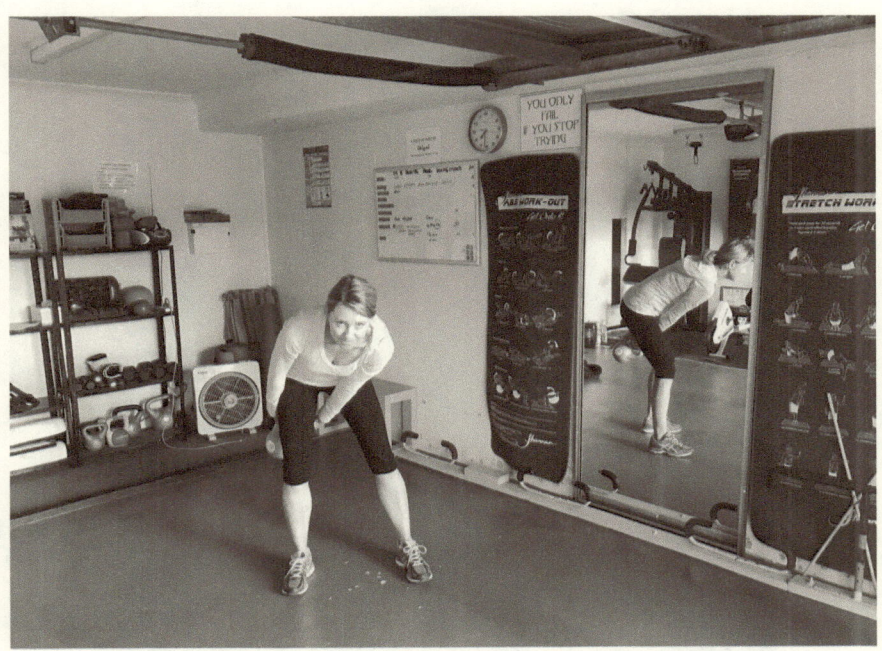

Here are my six kettlebell routines:

Routine 1

Standard moves: Complete standard moves one and two.

Exercise component: Dead lift

Place the kettlebell on the ground in front of you. Stand with your legs shoulder width apart. Bend your knees, squat, and grasp the bell with arms straight. Stand up holding the bell down with straight arms. Keeping your head up and your back straight, swing the bell back between your legs and then swing it up in the opposite direction over your head, keeping your arms straight.

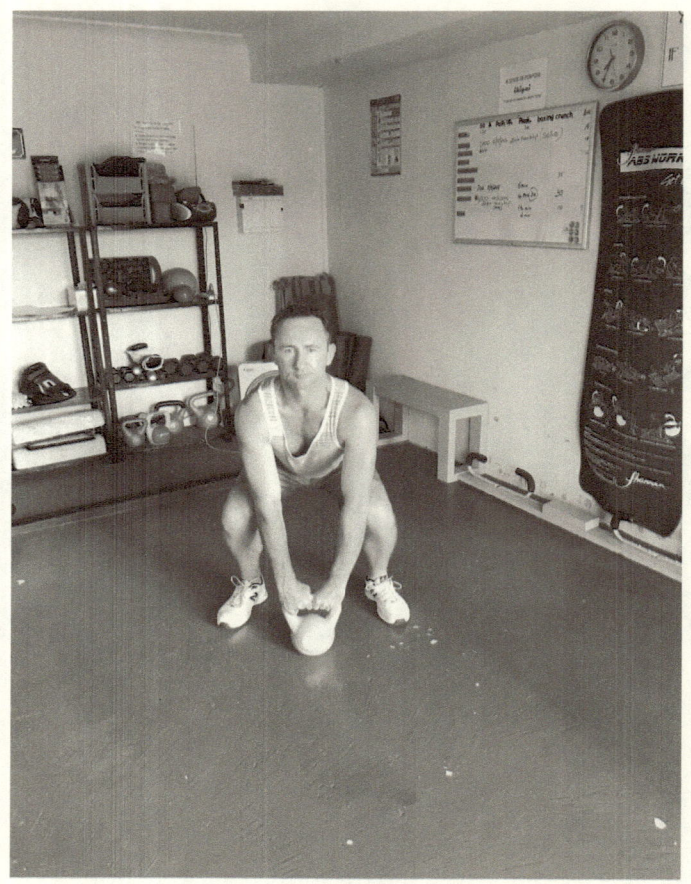

Routine 2

Standard moves: Complete standard moves one and two.

Exercise component: Squats

Stand upright and hold the kettlebell with both hands at your chest, elbows in near the body. Perform ten squats, keeping your head up, your heels in contact with the ground. Maintain a long spine—no drooping posture.

Routine 3

Standard moves: Complete standard moves one and two.

Exercise component: Wood chop

Stand upright with your feet at least shoulder width apart. Imagine your kettlebell is the head of an axe and your arms are the handle. You have a piece of wood between your feet which needs chopping. Swing with your arms straight out in front as you would in chopping a piece of wood with your head up and bent at the knees.

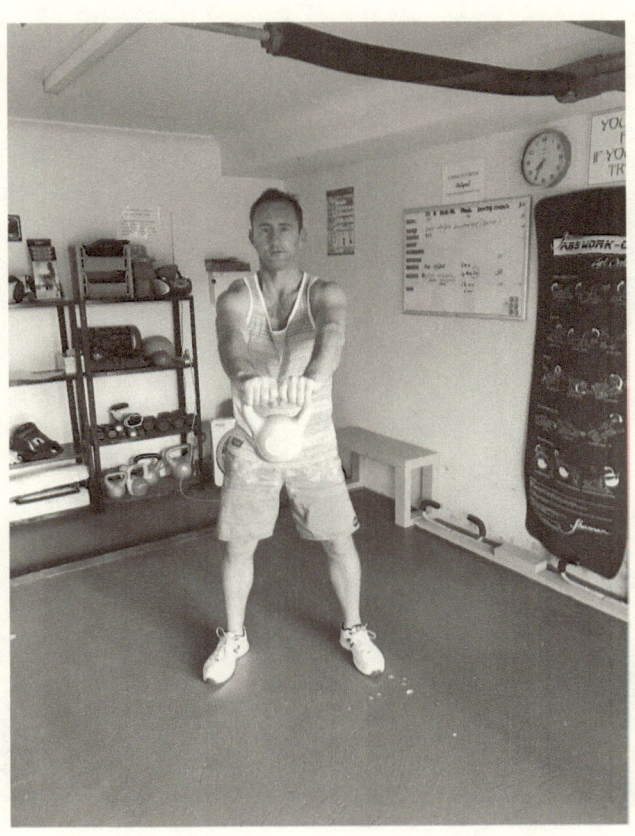

Routine 4

Standard moves: Complete standard moves one and two.

Exercise component: Overhead swing arch

Assume good standing posture and simply swing the kettlebell in an arch over the front of your head from one side of your body to the other starting at about waist height.

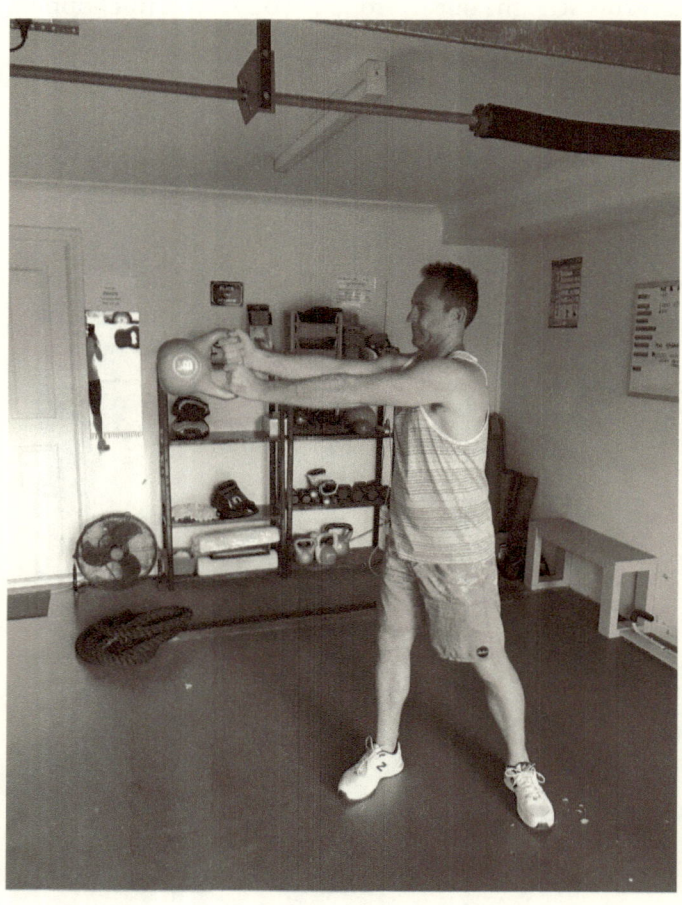

Routine 5

Standard moves: Complete standard moves one and two.

Exercise component: Lunge forward

Lunge or step forward with your right foot, then pass the kettlebell from one hand to the other under your bent right knee. Step back and repeat using your left leg, head up and back straight.

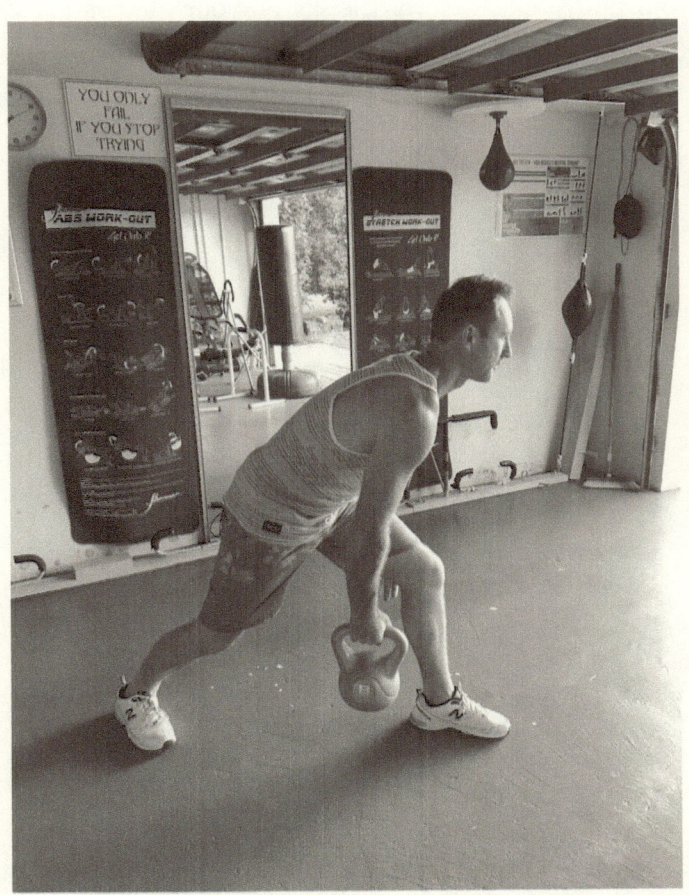

Routine 6

Standard moves: Complete standard moves one and two.

Exercise component: Low to high

Assume good standing posture and hold the kettlebell in your right hand. Perform a perfect squat, reaching down and touch your left foot with the kettlebell. When raising through the squat, bring the kettlebell across your body and reach for the sky on your right side. Repeat ten times then using your left hand and right foot repeat ten times.

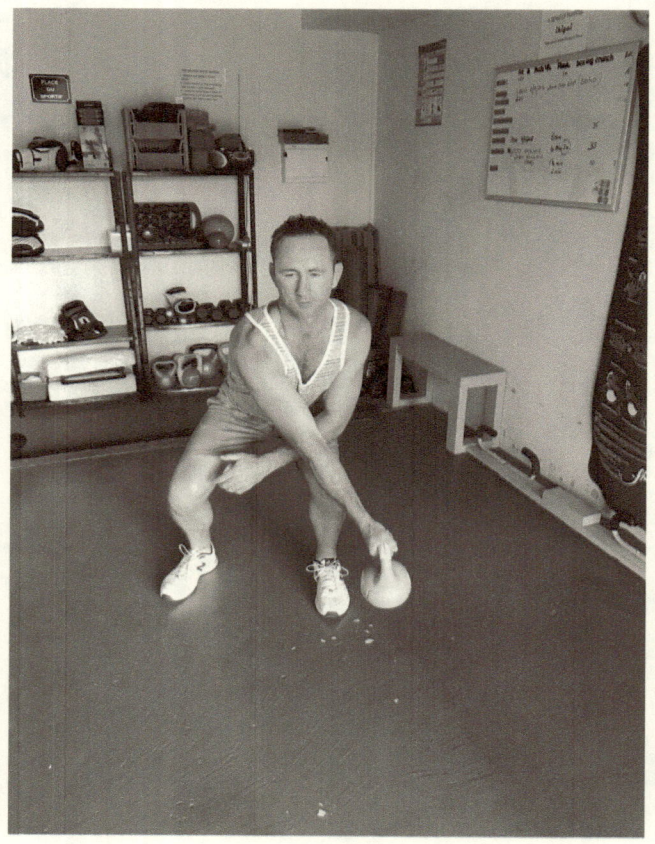

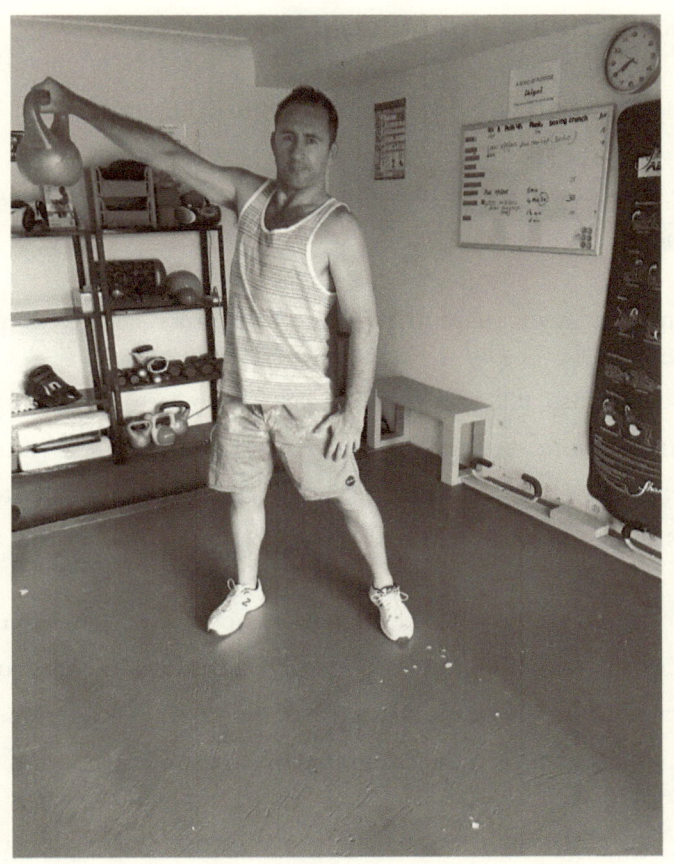

You can perform more difficult exercises with the kettlebell, but doing so could take away the free-flowing aerobic element and reduce some of the fun.

To quickly adapt the routines to a HISIART session, simply increase the intensity of the exercise component to bring your heart rate up. You can use the two standard moves as active rest to bring it down.

What kettlebell weight is right?

Petite, light-framed girl: 4 kilograms or 8 to 10 pounds

Average size female or small-framed man: 4 to 6 Kilograms or 13 to 15 pounds

Medium- to heavy-framed man: 6 to 8 kilograms or 15 to 20 pounds.

Some people may tell you these weights are not heavy enough for a strenuous workout, but that is not so. You will get great results with these weights. When you have finished fifteen to twenty minutes of my routines at a good pace, you will know it!

I have been working with kettlebells for over five years and I very rarely pick up an 8-kilogram bell (usually when it is the only one left). Consider this: an Olympic woman's shot put is 4 kilograms or 8.8 pounds, and a man's is 7.26 kilograms or just about 16 pounds.

I think you will find the weights I have recommended more than a challenge when used in a nonstop, fast-moving session.

Plenty of gain with no pain.

If you are time-poor and need to exercise wherever and whenever you can without equipment, read on.

Chapter 9

Your Body Can Be Your Gym

There are many exercises you can do using your own body weight. In my first book, I mentioned a lot of start-up exercises designed for beginners.

Start off with push-ups.

Push-ups are a perfect example, and you can begin by facing the wall and simply pushing yourself away from the wall. You can then advance to doing push-ups on your knees. Or on a set of stairs you can vary the level of strength required by placing your hands on different steps. The lower the step the more difficult it will be. Who cares if you never do a full push-up from the floor? Not everyone is physically developed or strong enough. I train a lot of aerobically fit women who have great, toned bodies and have no intention of building enough muscle mass to perform a standard push-up. In a standard push-up, you push your entire body weight away from gravity. You do not have to push yourself to the limit; all movement is good.

Move on to the plank.

There is one exercise that is gaining in popularity and should be included in your exercise routine. It can also be used as a replacement exercise for many other standard exercises you may be unable to do because of injuries. It can be done almost anywhere, anytime with no equipment necessary, just your own body weight. The benefits outweigh most other single exercises.The plank targets your core muscles to sculpt your waistline and improve your posture. Add a few variations and you can engage and build strength in your shoulders, back, glutes and hamstrings. The side plank work the obliques (your side abdominal muscle), which are not always targeted. All variations of the plank are great for improving flexibility and balance.

Here's how to my variation of the plank:

Some people perform the plank by supporting their straight bodies on their toes and elbows, forearms, and wrists. Others support their bodies on their toes and palms of the hands, like the "up" portion of a push up. I like to combine the two poses and add a side plank to make one great continuous exercise. Difficult? Yes! Do not expect to be able to perform the full routine straight off unless you are reasonably fit. It takes a period of time and bit of practice to perfect this routine.

Here's how to do it:

1. Start off in the standard plank position: toes and forearm supporting your weight as you keep your back and legs in a straight line. Hold the position for twenty seconds.

2. Move without relaxing to a side plank position: support your weight on the side of one foot and the forearm on the same side. Hold the

position for twenty seconds. Your upper arm can be full extended or placed on your hip.

3. Move back to the standard plank position; hold for twenty seconds.

4. Move into a side plank on the opposite side; hold for twenty seconds.

5. Return again to the standard plank position; hold for twenty seconds.

6. Finally, without relaxing, move to the push-up plank; hold for twenty seconds.

7. To finish the routine, stand up without relaxing and without your knees touching the floor.

The whole routine must be performed without relaxing and without support from any other body part except for those used in the plank position. If you are having trouble completing the full set of exercises without fault, practice lifting one leg when in the standard plank position to build and improve balance, strength, and muscle control.

Great core muscle gains, no pain!

If you have started a regular, consistent exercise routine, possibly one that lasts for one hour, and you do this three to four days a week, and if it is intense enough to be considered a hard workout (pushing yourself to increase your heart rate and experience some fatigue), *fantastic!* You have started to turn your life around. To maintain this lifestyle and avoid burnout, you are also going to need a break occasionally. Most sports people taper (reduce the amount of exercise) before an important event to freshen up so as they can give their best performance.

A lot of exercise or training programs work on an eight-week format: train hard for eight weeks then have a break. I prefer to work on a social-year calendar. To start with, the week between Christmas and the New Year is a perfect time for your first break. A day or two before or after the Easter break is another ideal time for a break. You can work school or work holidays into your schedule. When you are off on these breaks, you will feel great, and you will fully realise the enormous benefits you are gaining.

Chapter 10

Back Muscles: the Forgotten Group

What is one of the most important muscle areas of your body to strengthen with exercise?

Surprisingly, it is the back muscles. They are probably the most neglected, disregarded muscles because they are out of sight. Your arms, legs, and frontal core muscles make you look good. But the large group of muscles in your back support your spine, so what could be more important? Your back muscles protect the nerve centre of your body. This is the mechanism that conveys impulses to your brain. These muscles are also essential overall for good posture, balance, and core function. You may think sitting at a desk for extended periods of time is relatively easy on your back, but if you have poor posture, sitting in a hunched-over position for long periods without a break or a short walk or a few stretches can put a lot of pressure on your spine, and this can lead to back problems.

One of the most common types of chronic pain is back pain. Like any constant nagging pain, it can affect everything you do in life, including your mental performance, your memory, and your mood. Deficiencies in these areas add to the risk of anxiety and depression. If you can build up your back muscles to support your spine, you may prevent an injury, and if an injury does occur, strong muscles can lessen the severity of the injury and aid in recovery.

I do not have all the answers, but I may have one: good posture. This can be achieved with exercises that target your shoulders, back, and core. Integrated into your regular program, these exercises will go a long way in preventing painful back problems in the future. They may even relieve or cure existing problems, and that could remove a lot of distress and anxiety from your life.

There are many great back exercises you can do. I believe that the best one is the plank, which I have described in detail in the previous chapter. I keep repeating myself because it is so very beneficial, no equipment is necessary, and it can be done almost anywhere anytime. It is also harder than it looks, and it takes very little time. Because it is an isometric exercise, there is no movement involved, which means it has a low injury risk. Your muscles are working for and against each other to hold the position. Increase your endurance by slowly increasing the period you hold each of the steps before relaxing. Don't forget the side plank and raising your leg for even more balance, strength, and muscle control.

For a great overall muscle tone routine—including your back muscles— please refer to my chapter on kettlebells.

I said at the beginning of this chapter that our back muscles are often disregarded and neglected. Sometimes you might omit exercises that target your back or give them little importance in your session because they are out of sight. Well, out of sight to you maybe, but they are not to other people.

One of the women who comes to me for training was not overweight, just well covered and elegant yet she was still concerned about an unwanted layer of fat that seemed to be developing across her upper back. Some women call this "bra fat," and it is most obvious when wearing summer dresses and clothing made of clingy fabrics when it bulges out around bra bands and straps. She was prepared to work hard to avoid that look; she particularly wanted to look nice when she was dining out wearing some of her best dresses with low-cut backs. She was training with me for an hour every Monday, Wednesday, and Friday—a perfect schedule with a rest day in between sessions. I suggested that she should devote ten minutes of each session to upper back exercise. We were already doing a lot of abdominal exercises, which were building up her lower back around her love handle areas, but we needed to do a little for her upper back. We targeted that area with my full kettlebell routine, push-ups (most ladies perform push ups on their knees), and planks for about three months. One Monday morning she arrived at training all smiles. When I asked why she looked so happy, she told me she'd been trying on a bra in the changing cubical of a large department store over the weekend. There were mirrors on three of the four walls, and she was surprised when she actually saw how great her back looked. Now there is no stopping her!

To be motivated this way or to drop a dress size, or even find that your current wardrobe of clothes feels a bit loose beats a set of scales any day. Scales give you only a number. This body transformation is the real deal. It is something you can see and admire yourself, and other people can too. You can fix existing problem areas with exercise, and you can prevent the problems from developing in the first place. For this lady, it took a lot of discipline, willpower, foresight, and, of course, hard work to maintain and improve a body she was proud of. Some people maintain their motor vehicles to keep them running flawlessly at a "pride and joy" standard. Why not maintain your body to a similar standard so it becomes your pride and joy? It is not that hard—you can start by taking a walk.

A cure for a neglected body requires much more hard work, and it is difficult to turn things around, so change old habits and begin living a more active lifestyle. It all starts with your mindset—a mental framework of a positive attitude: "I can do this." To do nothing is to have complete disrespect for your body and how it functions. Like a motor vehicle, if it is not maintained correctly to a high standard, it will break down, and the cure will take a long time and will cost a lot. Prevention is quicker and cheaper!

If you are already overweight, you cannot target a particular localised fatty area like your upper back, belly, love handles, or any other part of your body. Unfortunately, it does not work that way. You have to reduce your overall body weight. Just doing sit-ups to improve your abdominal muscles will not reduce the fat in that area. You may end up with great abdominal muscles hidden under a layer of fat! Your body does not reduce fat levels in isolated areas. Any weight loss will be proportional.

Chapter 11

What Size Weights Should You Use?

Confused about what size weights to use to avoid injury, but still get a great result? Worry no more.

Here is an easy-to-understand guide for selecting the correct size weights for strength training, whether you are using free weights (hand weights), a bar with weights, or a machine. This guide fits all, and the recommended weights are ideal for toning and building muscle strength.

I won't list actual weights because the recommended weight can vary greatly depending on an individual's fitness level and frame sizes. If you are a light-framed person you will not be lifting the same weight a solid-built person would lift. Use this guide as a trial-and-error format to help you select the right weight for your body type. Always select a lighter weight to start and slowly increase the weight size as you gain fitness and muscle mass.

Level 1: This light weight feels easy. You experience free movement with no real effort. You may feel you could keep going for a long period, or you might feel that you need a heavier weight. It is better to use these light weights than to sit on the lounge.

Level 2: Some effort is required, but again, you feel you could keep going for a long period. This weight is great for beginners or people of mature age.

Level 3: A slight effort is required, and you feel a light tension in your muscles. This is ideal for beginners who are moving on.

Level 4: This weight is slightly heavier, but you still feel you can do quite a few reps. If you can do fifteen to twenty reps and find the last five are a little difficult, you have found the correct weight size for this stage. Continue with this weight until the last five reps are easy. Then increase the weight size.

Level 5: The weights feel quite heavy, but you have complete control. Only do a small number of reps. There is no need to push yourself until you feel physically fatigued.

If you can reach and maintain level 4 irrespective of weight size, in my view you will gain the most benefit.

Level 6: Once you have been training for a few months and have attained some fitness and muscle tone, use Level 4 80 per cent of the time and Level 5 20 per cent of the time. This is a great routine for bone density, on top of all the other great benefits.

If you are trying to improve yourself and lead a healthier lifestyle, exercise is only half the battle. What and how much you eat is of equal importance.

Chapter 12

Eating Habits

Grazing is the preferred option for a healthy body: small amounts consumed at regular intervals, rather than three big meals a day. The problem is that everything in our lives—work, rest, and play—is geared to three meals. Also, our minds are hardwired to three meals a day, and the time we consume them is regulated by the society we live in. So let us try a compromise to fit our eating habits to our modern lifestyle.

We can develop a grazing pattern but still maintain normal work and social guidelines. Let us make our three main meals smaller, still keeping them social and conforming. Add some quality health snacks in between. Fresh fruit is best. Try to reduce the window of time you are consuming your first and last meals of the day. You might have your first meal between six and seven in the morning and your last, say, between six and eight in the evening. Of course this may vary depending on your circumstances. What we are trying to achieve is a way of supplying your body with fuel for a slow release of energy for activities when it is most needed. We want to avoid a morning slump caused by little or no breakfast, or that sluggish wanting-to-have-a-nap feeling because your midday meal was too big and your energy is being used to digest food. You can also, as I mentioned in my first book, achieve an overnight mini fast by consuming water or tea only after you have finished your evening meal. Your next solid food intake would be the next morning at breakfast. What a great way to give your digestive system a break! It is easy to achieve, and best done during weekdays, so at weekends you can enjoy your social life.

At the moment maybe you have a light breakfast and rush off to work; a medium-sized lunch, sometimes while on the go; and a larger-sized meal at night.

Reverse your daily menu.

Try making your breakfast your larger-sized meal. You have not eaten for somewhere around ten hours, and you are going to need energy for your morning at work. It makes sense that this should be a meal that sustains you. Don't forget your fruit if you need it for midmorning snack. Lunch remains a medium-sized meal, and your evening meal can still be your main meal. Take time to consume it and socialise. Just make it a smaller meal as your energy expenditure and fuel requirement will both be smaller as you relax into the evening.

Your new healthy eating choices have to be enjoyable so they can be sustained long term. Choose healthy foods that you enjoy so you don't foresee an unpleasant experience or think that you will be living in denial. There are many great-tasting, common-sense choices you can make to achieve a well-balanced food intake. Lean meat, fish, fruit, vegetables, and wholegrain or sourdough bread are included. Eat foods that are as close to their natural state as possible. Try to avoid foods that have had too much human intervention such as processed or refined foods that contain added salt, sugar, and fats to increase sales volume.

Try to replace the word *diet*. Instead of saying you are "on a diet," say that you are "making healthy, common-sense eating choices." A diet suggests a temporary undertaking that lasts only until you achieve your desired goal. Then you go back to your old bad habits. Short-term weight loss will give you short-term, unsustainable results. Fad diets do not teach lasting, healthy eating habits.

Think of food as fuel for your body that is necessary for you to be able to do the miles during the day. Depriving your body of food by "dieting" will not give you that energy to do those miles. You will run out of energy. Grazing, on the other hand, will give you a slow, long-lasting, steady release of fuel. You do not overfill your car with fuel, so do not over eat. You do not let your car run out of fuel, so don't deprive your body.

Denying yourself food when you are "dieting" will burn some fat reserves, but is it sustainable? Or does it lead to the yo-yo effect: periods of excessive indulgence (binging) followed by starving yourself.

The same healthy eating choices do not fit or work the same for everyone; we are all different. A twenty-five-year-old male with a big frame who works hard in a manual-type job will have different requirements to a fifty-year-old light-framed male and a petite female who work sitting at a desk most days.

Dieting can also be dangerous. Being thin does not necessarily mean you are healthy. Because you think thin is good, you may not realise you have a health problem. You may lack muscle mass, flexibility, and fitness, and you could still have hidden fat on the inside around your vital organs. Unhealthy thin people with low muscle mass run similar risks of developing diabetes as people who are overweight. Do not compromise healthy behaviour just to be thin. Say a big "no" to crash dieting. These plans are not healthy and very rarely work. They do not always increase your metabolism. Your body can go into starvation mode, and your metabolic rate can decrease, and this lessens your possibilities for quick weight loss. You may start to lose some of your lean muscle as your body senses a problem and starts to hold onto fat to help you survive.

The big three to avoid or reduce for healthy eating: sugar, salt, and fats.

Sugar

Not all sugar is harmful to your health. You need sugar in your blood; it can supply you with a large amount of energy. Unfortunately, sugar contains few essential nutrients, and if consumed to excess, it is seriously harmful.

We may be conscientious and regulate the amount of sugar we add to coffee, tea, or breakfast cereal, or we may leave it out altogether. Yet we fail to check for sugar hidden in the processed foods that contributes a high percentage to our average daily intake. We may also be alert to the fact that most soft drinks are loaded with sugar, but blind to the fact most fruit juices, cereals, a wide range of processed meat, and some yoghurts have added sugar.

Many so-called healthy processed products contain sugar. Check the labels; sugar can be disguised as glucose, fructose, sucrose, high-fructose corn syrup, or any ingredient ending in the letters *ose*.

One teaspoon of sugar = 4.2 grams = 16 calories. Adding sugar to your diet from whole fruit is best. Sugar from overly processed savoury food is bad.

Salt

We all need salt in our bodies to help regulate fluid levels, but there is generally more than enough in a normal diet without adding anymore. The recommendation for salt intake is no more than four to six grams a day for adults. That equals approximately one teaspoon. How do you know how much salt you are consuming? It is very difficult to know because most bread, cereals, and processed food have salt added, as it is a great flavour enhancer. If you can cut down on fast and take-away foods, stop adding salt to your food at home, and check the nutrition labels on pre-packaged food, you will be doing yourself a big favour. You will be going a long way in reducing your salt intake and greatly reducing your chances of having heart problems in the future.

Here is a quick guide for checking labels. Some labels list salt as sodium:

> Salt: 1.5 grams of salt per 100 grams of food product is high.

> Sodium: 0.6 grams of sodium per 100 grams of food product is high.

Put the high-salt, high-sodium products back on the shelf and select a product with a lower ratio.

Fats

Much of what we eat contains fat. As it is with salt, it is essential to have some fat in your diet, although having too much is harmful to your health. There are good fats, not so bad fats, and bad fats.

You may think the fat in juicy steak or a piece of chicken (skin off) eaten in moderation is great, and it is, but there are better fats like the healthy, unsaturated fats found in fish, nuts, and seeds. But even these good fats, if eaten in large quantities, will contribute to weight gain. So, once again, everything in moderation. You can also spoil the goodness of your red meat, fish, or poultry by deep-frying in refined vegetable oil. This will add unhealthy trans-fats (bad fats). It is much healthier to pan fry in a small amount of extra virgin olive oil. Or better still, use a grill so fats drain away.

I hate to be a killjoy, but a lot of your favourite processed foods contain trans-fats: cakes, biscuits, cookies, crackers, frozen pizza crusts, and more. The trans-fats in these foods provide a good-looking texture plus a desirable taste, which sell the manufacturers' products.

Always, if possible, check the nutrition or ingredient list panel on the packaging for trans-fats or partially hydrogen oil. Zero is best.

Try to limit how often you eat these products; possibly have them as a special treat.

Don't cut out fat; replace bad fat with good fat.

> ***Good fat:*** Unsaturated fats (monounsaturated fatty acids)
>
> *Main source:* Fish, lean meat, nuts and seeds all in sensible size portions and as a treat peanut butter.
>
> *Tip:* Still eat in moderation and, on your plate, make these the small portion. The large portion should be vegetables or salad.

Okay fat: Saturated fats. (limited intake advised)

Main source: All animal products, including fatty meats, butter, cheese, eggs etc.

Tip: Eat less of these.

Bad fats. Trans-fats (partially hydrogenated oils)

Main source: Commercially baked goods and packaged foods.

Tip: Avoid these foods because they can lower good cholesterol and raise bad cholesterol.

Do a food swap.

Red meat.

It's best not to eat red meat every day.

Swap to: Lean cuts of red meat twice a week, then swap to chicken, turkey (no skin on either), eggs, and fish.

Fruit juices.

These are usually low in fibre high in sugar.

Swap to: Whole fruits contain good sugar and great fibre, and they come in their own natural packaging.

Cereals.

Unless you pick a good one, they can contain anything except what is good for you.

Swap to: Oats (cooked oatmeal) provide great fibre and give you that full feeling for longer, which can curb unhealthy snacking.

Low fat yoghurt.

Low fat can mean high sugar content for better flavour.

Swap to: Greek yoghurt, a good source of calcium and low in sugar.

Muesli and energy bars.

These are highly processed, low in nutrients, and packed with sugar.

Swap to: Whole fruit. All fruit is great—bananas are most favoured by sports people for extra energy.

Processed Foods.

Fats, sugar, and salt are all added for taste to increase sales.

Swap to: Fruit, vegetables, and eggs. These are all natural foods, fresh from the farm.

It is not always about what you eat, it's sometimes about how much you eat and also what you don't eat.

The wrong foods, especially if you consume them in excessive amounts, can be poison.

The right foods consumed in moderate amounts can be medicine.

Here's a note about honey: Even though honey has a high percentage of sugar, I believe a small amount consumed on most days provides some natural health benefits.

Chapter 13

Think Before You Eat

With your new lifestyle changes, for a short period of time you may have to think before you eat. You will be changing some deeply rooted ingrained habits and fighting against addictive foods—highly processed foods, and fast and take-away foods, all of which contain added salt, sugar, and fats. You may even be accustomed to adding too much salt and sugar to your home-cooked meals. Even the way you cook can be addictive. So don't go cold turkey.

As you do when starting an exercise program, make small changes gradually. Moving forward with a series of changes gives your body, particularly your taste buds, time to adjust. My favourite food is fresh bread. I love it, even to the point of mild addiction, so I still have my fresh bread. I just don't have it every day. When you go on a fad/crash diet, your body is denied food at a radical rate. This extreme change causes your body to go into shock. Your body begins to cannibalise itself. You do lose fat and weight, but because your body is in conflict with itself, your general health is at risk.

With common sense as your guide, and knowing that crash diets cannot be good for your body, you will want to do something similar at a much slower, consistent rate to achieve a sustainable, realistic goal. Create great habits that will last a lifetime and will develop a body to be proud of—one in which you can live and enjoy the world.

A quick, easy, general rule for a safe sustainable weight loss guide is to lose as little as half a kilogram, or one pound, a week or less. Be patient and look at the long-term picture.

Weight loss can be hard work, and when we look at a meal we are about to eat or even a snack, we may tend to underestimate how much energy and vigorous activity we need to burn off what we are about to consume. So you can appreciate and fully understand the challenge before you, here is an example how much work is required to burn of fat/weight:

> A thirty-minute light jog will burn 120 calories. Most hamburgers start at 350 calories, and these are the good ones.

> You would have to jog for one hour to burn off a cup of coffee and a muffin.

So, do the figures before you eat!

We have covered exercise, sleep, and eating habits as being very important. You should also consider rest and relaxation. Some people are guilty of too much; others of not enough.

Chapter 14

Recovery Session after a Hard Day at Work

You arrive home after a hard stressful day at work. Possibly you have been sitting all day with bad posture. Possibly your day was filled with lots of drama. I worked for the last twenty-four years before I retired at age sixty-five with the emergency automotive roadside assistance patrol. I spent most of each day driving in traffic and dealing with the occasional stressful situation—a baby locked in a car on a hot day or a breakdown in a dangerous location.

The first thing you want to do when you arrive home is to grab a beer or a glass of wine, crash on the lounge, and flick on the television. What is the first thing to come on? The nightly news, filled with drama—just what you do not need after a stressful day.

Try a different approach. I did, and it works. As soon as you walk in your front door, have a drink of water, change your clothes if you need to, and go for a thirty-minute walk. Take your partner, friend, or dog. Hold your head up and keep your shoulders back. Walk tall. You are switching off and walking out and away from the stresses of the day, clearing your head, taking in the sights and sounds around you.

What a great way to connect and think about—and perhaps discuss—the day's events without any distractions. You will return home refreshed both mentally and physically. Again, have a glass of water; this time make it a large one.

You may find you do not need the beer, wine, or spirits. If you still choose to have some, most likely you will be able to sit down with better posture, drink your beverage slowly, and enjoy it more.

Throwing yourself on the lounge with a six-pack of beer does not work. You will not sleep as deeply in the night as you should, and you will wake the next morning ill prepared for the day ahead because your brain will be in a fog. With significantly hindered alertness and mental performance, you will be open to making mistakes. Rather, if you follow my advice, you can wake up with a clear head, without that morning grogginess. You'll feel energised and ready for the day ahead. This could be the start of a lifesaving exercise habit. At the very least you will gain the benefits of relaxed incidental exercise.

Many gains and no pain.

If you have a job that follows you around 24/7, take a tip: when you go for a recovery session walk, leave your mobile phone at home and give yourself time to think – it can work wonders It is incredible how many problems you can solve when you have a clear head, and when you have no voices coming at you from every direction. My job as a motor mechanic was reasonably uncomplicated but still very important. (I say uncomplicated because only those in a management role had to deal with unpredictable human emotions; for the rest of us, the job did not involve thinking outside the square.) In my job, there were no grey areas. There was a reason for every problem, and if I could eliminate any mental pressure and think the problem through in an orderly manner, I could then find and solve the problem.

Many times I have gone to bed at night with a problem on my mind and awakened in the morning with the answer. Things seem to come into your mind when your brain is not cluttered and confused with too much information.

Give yourself space and time for your training to kick in.

Most of this book was first written in my mind whilst I was on one of my many long casual walks. If I repeat myself and present a life-changing thought or idea more than once, that's okay, as it must be important enough to bear repeating. It will be something you should remember every day, and it is what I believe in most strongly.

I want these lifestyle changes etched in your mind 24/7 so you accept them as a commonplace part of your normal routine without having to think about them. You don't have to become a health fanatic; you just have to make a few sensible compromises.

Take a Break

Chapter 15

If You Take Nothing Else from My Book, Remember This:

- Everything starts with a positive mind; your body and mind should complement each other and work as one.

- Your mindset must be resilient so you can bounce back after any setback.

- Don't sit around counting the days. Make as many days count as you possibly can.

- If you are too lazy to get off the lounge and move now, one day you may be denied the pleasure.

- Movement is a gift. Just ask people who can't move. Do not be diverted or distracted from consciously focusing on what you can do.

- Are you hungry or bored? If you answer yes to bored, go for a walk.

- If you are hungry but do not really need food, and you're not bored, have a glass of water. Don't indulge in emotional eating. Ask yourself, "Do I really need to eat the whole chocolate block or packet of biscuits? Or would one biscuit or one piece of chocolate satisfy me just as well?"

- You need to remove temptation. What you don't see you don't necessarily crave.

- The improved muscle tone, fitness, and balance you gain from exercise will enhance your ability to perform your normal daily routine.

- Move more; eat less. The more you move, the less you are inclined to eat.

- Everything in moderation. You can still have a great life; just use some restraint and don't go to extremes—reduce the excessiveness of some of your eating and drinking habits. I use the 80/20 policy: For 80 per cent of the time (usually weekdays), I try to eat well and exercise. And for 20 per cent of the time (weekends), I relax and enjoy.

- All movement is good.

- Limit your intake of processed foods. I know they are easy, but fresh is always best.

- Fast food is a treat and should be treated as such; it is not part of a well-balanced diet.

- Always try to have something to look forward too, even if it is only something small or simple.

- Make exercise fun. Once you have gained some fitness and you start to enjoy exercise, you will automatically tend to start to eat better and eat less.

- If you are having problems getting started, seek help. Most people need a bit of help.

- Don't worry about what other people think. Don't listen to their criticism. They are the negative ones living in denial.

- Practice good posture 24/7. It is not as hard as it sounds, and it will soon become second nature.

- Eating habits should be common sense—no fad diets. Look for an overall balanced way of eating.

- Don't add salt or sugar. Limit your fat intake.

- Any extra movement is good, especially if it is more than you are doing now.

- Being lean and fit won't distract from your social life. It will improve it 100 per cent. You will look great while still being able to enjoy having a few social drinks and eating sensibly.

- When doing exercise, activity, or movement, try to make it intense enough to increase your heart rate.

- Sometimes the simplest exercises are the most beneficial, and you don't need any fancy machines.

- Don't let trivial things rule your life and define who you are. Remember to exercise your brain as well as your body.

- What defines us from other species on this earth (God-given maybe) is the strong urge to be better. These characteristics are built into every one of us; you just need a change of attitude and a positive mind to bring it out.

- Don't give yourself time to hesitate, overthink your situation, or find an excuse for not exercising and eating well.

- Now is the time! No more procrastination! Get up off the lounge and go for a walk. It is that simple. Just as you have started most journeys in life, start with one small step.

Moving forward – no pain.

Chapter 16

Incidental Exercise

If, even after reading my book, you are still having trouble finding the time or motivation for exercise, and if you are still leading a sedentary lifestyle and baulk at the concept of a life-changing fitness and weight loss program, at least, as a last resort, try incidental exercise.

Incidental exercise is any robust, vigorous, or energetic activity that is part of the routine of your everyday life; it is "built-in activity." This could be something you would normally take for granted, like playing with your children or grandchildren, walking the dog, washing the car, or any number of activities. You can always do these things with more enthusiasm. Some people say that playing a round of golf spoils a good walk. That walk (and that golf swing!) could keep you young.

You can also make a lot of life style changes, such as doing your own washing, ironing, and cleaning instead of employing someone. Walk and perform squats while talking on the phone. Squats are a neglected fundamental movement. You performed them over and over as a child. It is a very natural movement, and it works a lot of muscles including your abs and lower back, not just your legs. It is easy on your joints, and if performed frequently, can replace a walk or jog. Squats will improve your thighs, hips, and glutes (backside), and will also help to keep your legs in shape.

Here is the correct way to do a squat:

> You can build up to this exercise by using a chair, and then transition to no chair. Stand with your feet the same distance apart as your hips. Form a straight line between your toes, knees, and hips. Engage your abs and slowly lower your body, keeping long in the spine, just as if you were lowering yourself onto a chair. Go as low as you can while still feeling confident you can raise your body back up. With your head up, drive your body back up through your heels. Keep practising until your knees form a right angle or lower. If you have trouble keeping your balance when you are not using a chair, extend your hands out to the front while focusing on an object that is directly in front of you.

Tips:

- Don't make any side movement; go straight up and down.

- Stay long in the spine—no hunching.

- Keep your head up and keep looking forward.

- Always keep your heel in contact with floor.

- Draw your belly button to your spine.

- Keep your knees "soft" (slightly bent) at top of movement.

- Breathe in on the down movement and out as you drive back up.

- Extend arms forward for balance.

- Check your form by looking at a mirror that is off to your side.

Of course the best two life changes, when possible, are to leave your car at home and walk to work, the train, the bus, the shops, and to use the stairs whenever you can instead of taking the lift. You should do more, but even these small changes will be a start.

Moderate gain, no pain.

Chapter 17

Conclusion

I am not trying to introduce anything new—no extreme exercise regimes, no detoxing, no fasting, no drinking only water for twenty-four hours, no radical diets.

In fact, as I have mentioned, I do not like the word *diet* when it refers to or implies a short-term change or fix before you go back to your old bad habits. Your body responds and performs much better to consistent, long-term care rather than forced crash and burn with sporadic treatments or short-term fad diets. Learn to say no to unhealthy food even when it is offered by a friend. You cannot please everyone. Do not skip meals; your body needs food for energy. Eat until you satisfied, not full. It is all about common sense. You do not need a dietician to inform you that you have bad eating habits. We hear about the twentieth- and twenty-first century obesity problem frequently on the news.

Living to an old age with a good quality of life is your birthright. Do not throw it away. Get the most out of your life. Do not get old before your time—old age will come soon enough! Life is already too short. If you are currently living a sedentary lifestyle sitting in a chair most days, that chair you are sitting in could be a killer. Do not sit back and accept a life of premature decline and discomfort. Do not give in to being someone you don't wish to be! Create a life you want to live in, not a life you feel you need a holiday from.

Without some exercise or regular activity, your body will inevitably deteriorate. If you do not make an effort and put aside time now to look after your health, you may be forced to make time later in life to address and treat health problems that can be traced back to an inactive lifestyle. Carrying too much weight (body fat) over a long period of time causes many serious but avoidable chronic (long-lasting) conditions. Type 2 diabetes is a perfect example, but a high percentage of those at risk can prevent the onset by making lifestyle changes *now!*

I often think about the indigenous people who lived in America, Canada, Australia, and New Zealand before Europeans arrived. They lived in complete harmony with the land, only taking what they needed each day to survive. They held the land and animals as sacred. Their religion and culture revolved around living as one and having respect for nature, a lifestyle that was completely sustainable. I am also conscious how modern man has made advances in medicine and technology— advantages I certainly would not want to be without. We enjoy comforts that were unheard of or only dreamt about one hundred years ago. And they may not necessarily be sustainable. Wouldn't it be great if we could somehow marry the two philosophies and develop a compromise that would help reduce the rate of global warming and our obesity epidemic, two of the biggest challenges we have today?

We are looking for a win/win situation. One of the most obvious is to leave your car at home and walk wherever possible. Your car does not pollute the air unless it is driven, and your body gets the healthy benefit of use. Use the stairs and not the lift. Eat less food, particularly if it is processed. All of these suggestions may make only a small difference, but if every person joined in, what a huge difference it would make.

You put on the weight slowly over many years, and you have grown used to it. You think this is normal. You look around and see others of a similar weight, and this convinces or at least persuades you that everything is okay. *Wrong!* We are slowly becoming immobile as a species. You have that extra weight on your body 24/7. Imagine the extra unnecessary stress you are putting on your body. I see a lot of middle-aged people who are obese and need a cane to support and assist them when walking. I can't help but think that, for most of them, it is a case of "lose the weight and lose the cane."

If you observe people who are not overweight, you will see how much extra energy they have. Additionally, they experience ease and wide range of movement.

Like most things in life, getting started is the hardest part. Once you begin, things seem to fall into place, and you keep moving on. You do not have to lead a Spartan or frugal lifestyle, constantly denying yourself small pleasures in life. Just do not overindulge in eating and drinking to excess. And increase your physical activity. Anything new is a challenge! Once you do get started, do not set your goal too high. You can always set new ones after you achieve your first one. And, after you have set your goal, break it down into stages. Do not try to run the race in one hit; rather, tackle each hurdle as it presents itself, then move on to tackle the next one.

As I have previously mentioned, your mindset is incredibly important. If you have a positive mindset and believe you can achieve your goal, you will. If you have a negative mindset and lack confidence, and you don't believe in your own abilities, you won't. Positive people challenge themselves while knowing their limits.

Negative people underestimate their own ability and will not challenge themselves. If you are currently a negative person lacking in confidence and drive, I hope this book will help change your mindset, because more often than not, that is all that is required to turn your life around.

How crazy is it that a serious condition—type 2 diabetes—has become a modern-day lifestyle curse as most people are not born with it and it's not passed on by infection, it is self inflicted! Our bad, lazy lifestyle is damaging our blood vessels and, with time, will substantially affect so many parts of our bodies, including eyes, brain, kidney, heart, limbs, even our nervous system. And all of this is completely *avoidable*. The prevention is similar to the management.

Prevention is the only answer: Lead a healthy, active lifestyle and eat food that is as natural as possible. Practice moderation in everything you do. A good indicator of your general health is your waist measurement. This is measured at the narrowest part of your torso, usually just above your belly button. Regardless of your height, women should measure less than thirty-two inches (eighty-one centimetres), and men should measure less than thirty-eight inches (ninety-six centimetres). Anything above these measurements, and you are putting your health at risk.

The cause of overweight and obesity? It's simple: lack of physical activity combined with too much of an unhealthy diet that includes excess fat, salt, and sugar.

Management and possible cure: Eat less and switch to a healthier diet. Cut out or reduce processed foods with their added salt, sugar, and fat.

You must add physical activity to your lifestyle making small, and in some cases large, changes and sticking to them long term. This could save you from having to make more difficult lifesaving changes in years to come.

The solution, as I have explained, is very simple, so keep that way. Don't keep constantly reinventing new ways or be swayed by new fad diets or new fat-blasting routines or machines.

Changes now can save you future pain.
Be the best person you can be.

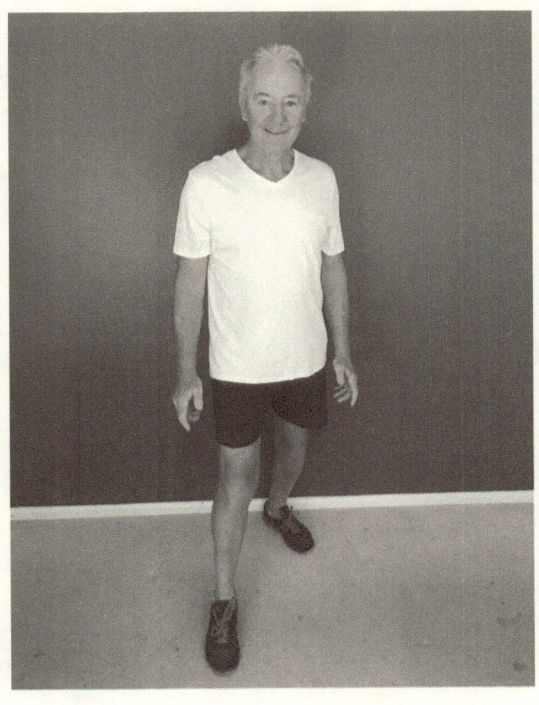

Do not become a prisoner in your own body.

If you are overweight, if your mobility is restricted and your lifestyle confined because of obesity, you can turn it around. Seek help if need be. You may need help, because it won't be easy. Anyone who tells you different is lying. It will take a lot of hard work that only you can do, but the rewards will far outweigh any sacrifices.

Set yourself free.
Start now.